Anti-Inflammatory Diet for Beginners

The complete guide to Lose Weight and Reduce Inflammation with 2000 days of Recipes and 61 Day Meal Plan

By

Adam Bennet

© **Copyright 2022 by Adam Bennet- All rights reserved.**

This document is geared towards providing exact and reliable information in regard to the topic and issue covered. The publication is sold with the idea that the publisher is not required to render accounting, officially permitted, or otherwise, qualified services. If advice is necessary, legal, or professional, a practiced individual in the profession should be ordered.

From a Declaration of Principles, which was accepted and approved equally by a Committee of the American Bar Association and a Committee of Publishers and Associations.

In no way is it legal to reproduce, duplicate, or transmit any part of this document in either electronic means or in printed format. Recording of this publication is strictly prohibited, and any storage of this document is not allowed unless with written permission from the publisher. All rights reserved.

The information provided herein is stated to be truthful and consistent, in that any liability, in terms of inattention or otherwise, by any usage or abuse of any policies, processes, or directions contained within is the solitary and utter responsibility of the recipient reader. Under no circumstances will any legal responsibility or blame be held against the publisher for any reparation, damages, or monetary loss due to the information herein, either directly or indirectly.

Respective authors own all copyrights not held by the publisher.

The information herein is offered for informational purposes solely and is universal as so. The presentation of the information is without contract or any type of guaranteed assurance.

The trademarks that are used are without any consent, and the publication of the trademark is without permission or backing by the trademark owner. All trademarks and brands within this book are for clarifying purposes only and are owned by the owners themselves, not affiliated with this document.

Disclaimer

We hope you enjoy the inspired and fun recipes written in our book. We are not responsible for the outcome of any recipe you try from this book. You may not achieve desired results due to variations in elements such as ingredients, cooking temperatures, typos, errors, omissions, or individual cooking ability. You should always use your best judgment when cooking with raw ingredients and seek expert advice before beginning if you are unsure. You should always take care when using sharp knives or other cooking implements. To ensure the safety of yourself and others, be aware of heated cooking surfaces while cooking. Please review all ingredients prior to trying a recipe to be fully aware of the presence of substances which might cause an adverse reaction in some consumers. Recipes available in the book may not have been formally tested by us or for us and we do not provide any assurances nor accept any responsibility or liability regarding their originality, quality, nutritional value, or safety. Unless otherwise stated, the recipes written in this book are not endorsed by any other companies/organization or their affiliates.

Contents

Introduction 9

Chapter 1: Anti-inflammatory Diet - What to know? 11

    1.1 *What is an anti-inflammatory diet?* 11

    1.2 *Types of an anti-inflammatory diet* 12

    1.3 *Who can it help?* 12

    1.4 *Foods to eat* 13

    1.5 *Foods to Avoid* 14

    1.6 *Can a vegetarian diet reduce inflammation?* 15

    1.7 *Anti-inflammatory diet tips* 15

    1.8 *Takeaway* 16

    1.9 *11 Ways to Make the Most of An Anti-Inflammatory Diet + A Food List* 16

    1.10 *Anti-inflammatory diet tips.* 16

    1.11 *Best anti-inflammatory food list.* 18

    1.12 *Foods to avoid on an anti-inflammatory diet.* 20

    1.13 *61 Days Diet Plan* 21

Chapter 2: Breakfast recipes 34

    1. *Quinoa Porridge with Chai-Infused Vanilla* 34

    2. *Power shake (alkaline avocado)* 35

    3. *Quinoa bread* 36

    4. *Basil overnight stone fruit oats* 37

    5. *Tropical Overnight Chia and Oats* 37

    6. *Chia Pudding with Layered Coconut Spirulina* 38

    7. *Detox Green Smoothie Monster* 39

    8. *Detox Porridge with Whipped Berry* 40

    9. *Acai Breakfast Bowl* 41

    10. *Kale Tapenade, Toast, and Avocado* 41

    11. *Grain, Nut & Gluten-Free Muesli* 42

    12. *Mango Mint Smoothie Bowl* 43

    13. *West Coast Avocado Toast* 43

    14. *Chia Pudding* 44

    15. *Fruit salad* 45

    16. *Pecans with roasted pears* 46

17. Berry Blast Porridge 47
18. Cycling Balls of Seed 48
19. Turmeric Tea with Golden Milk 48
20. Beet Smoothie for Immune Strengthening 49
21. Grapefruit and Blood Orange Salad with Cinnamon 50
22. Chili Relleno Casserole 51
23. Breakfast Salad with Salsa Verde Vinaigrette 52
24. Breakfast Potatoes 52
25. Camp Breakfast 53
26. Breakfast Strata 54
27. Superfood Breakfast 55
28. Breakfast Pasta 56
29. Breakfast Wellington 57
30. Avocado & Kale Omelet 58
31. Transition Breakfast Muesli 59
32. Alkaline Fibre Muesli 60
33. Seedy Breakfast 60
34. Alkaline Bean Salsa Baked Brekkie 61
35. scrambled Tofu & Tomato Brekkie 62
36. California Breakfast Salad 63

Chapter 3: Lunch Recipes 65
1. "Heart-Friendly" Salsa 65
2. Mushroom Risotto 66
3. Raw Energy Balls 66
4. Alkaline Wraps 67
5. Avocado Couscous Salad Recipe 68
6. Chunky English Garden Salad Recipe 69
7. Sunrise Turmeric Tonic 70
8. Detox Wrap with Sunflower Seed Spread 70
9. Spaghetti Squash Hash Browns 71
10. Roasted Vegetable Salad for Hormone Balance 72
11. Thai Cauliflower Rice Salad with Peanut Butter Sauce 73
12. Tabbouleh 75
13. Vegetable stew 76

14. Bliss Balls 77
15. Raw Cacao Energy Balls 78
16. Quinoa Bowl with Lentils and Mustard Vinaigrette 79
17. Perfectly Roasted Sweet Potato Fries 80
18. Split Pea Soup with Coconut (Spiced) 81
19. Miso-Harissa Delicate Squash And Brussels Sprouts Salad 83
20. One-Pot Curried Cauliflower with Couscous and Chickpeas 84
21. Grain Bowl with Spiced Squash & Mushrooms 85
22. Mediterranean Quinoa Salad with Roasted Veggies 86
23. Cinnamon Carrot Sticks 88
24. Foolproof Spinach & Feta Frittata 88
25. Lentil, Beetroot, & Hazelnut Salad along with Ginger Dressing 89
26. Tofu Curry 90
27. Easy and Yummiest Kulfi Recipe 91
28. Guacamole 91
29. Homemade Lunch Combination 92

Chapter 4: Dinner Recipes 93
1. Portobello mushroom burgers 93
2. Magic green falafels 94
3. Roast tomato and orange soup recipe 95
4. Green Detox Smoothie Bowl 96
5. Alkaline Lasagne 97
6. Kale Detox Salad with Pesto 98
7. Detox rainbow roll-ups with peanut sauce 100
8. Comforting Cashew Curry 101
9. Spicy Carrot & Greens 102
10. Roasted Cauliflower Detox Bowl with Tahini Sauce 102
11. Easy Veggie Wrap with Avocado and Halloumi 104
12. Seven-veg stir-fry 20 105
13. Alkaline Cous-Cous 107
14. Thai Green Curry Made Alkaline 107
15. Alkaline Lunchtime Wraps 109
16. Kale Slaw & Creamy Dressing 110
17. GABA rice + a Mental-Health Supporting Bowl 111

18. Aubergine & black bean Alkaline Chili 112
19. Stir-fry mushroom and broccoli 113
20. Grilled mackerel with chili, orange, lemon, and watercress 114
21. Quick Orecchiette Pasta with Kale Pesto 115
22. Vegetarian Pizza with Autumn Toppings 116
23. Spicy Kimchi Tofu Stew 118
24. Alkaline Chili non-Carne 119
25. Tomato Pie with Honey 120
26. Black Bean Quinoa Burger with Activated Charcoal Bun 121
27. Lentil Pasta with Kale and Marinara Sauce 123
28. Joseph's Best Easy Bacon Recipe 124
29. Alkaline Veggie Fajitas 125
30. Aubergine & Chickpeas Balti 126
31. Roasted cauliflower, fennel, and ginger soup 127
32. Easy Kielbasa Skillet Dinner 128
33. Easy Dinner Hash 129
34. Classic Carrot & Coriander Soup 130
35. Hobo Dinner 131
36. New Year's Day Dinner 131
37. Autumn Tomato & Avocado Warmer 132
38. Alkaline Gazpacho 133
39. Chopped Veggie Grain Bowls with Turmeric Dressing 134
40. Alkaline Raw Soup 134
41. Kale & Avocado Salad with Blueberries & Edamame 135
42. Alkaline Tom Yum Soup 136

Chapter 5: Snacks and Appetizers 138
1. Fruit Race Cars for Kids 138
2. Hot garlic ginger Lemonade 139
3. The Ginger Shot That Will Keep Cold and Flu Away 140
4. Turmeric, ginger, & lemon shots 141
5. Ginger Lemon Immune Boosting Shots 141
6. Pineapple turmeric sauerkraut and gut shots 142
7. How to make probiotic-rich water kefir 143
8. Vanilla bean and honey kefir panna cotta 144

9. Lemon verbena kombucha 145
10. Ginger beet sauerkraut 146
11. Jalapeno cilantro sauerkraut 147
12. Homemade Kimchi 148
13. Healthy homemade lemonade (naturally sweetened) 150
14. Avocado and Herb Salad 151
15. All-natural tamarind paste 152
16. Tea Recipe Five Flavored Autumn 152
17. Psyllium Apple & Lemon Balm Tea 153
18. Immunity-boosting soup 153
19. Nori-burritos 154
20. Cucumber basil gazpacho 155
21. Dandelion strawberry salad 156
22. Carrot & Courgetti Stack 157
23. Matcha Green Tea Latte 158
24. Winter Kale & Quinoa Salad with Avocado 158
25. Spiced Pecans 159
26. Warm Lentil salad 160
27. Herbal Chamomile Health Tonic 161
28. Coleslaw Zing 162
29. Broad Beans Salad with Turmeric Tomatoes 163
30. Crispy Roasted Chickpeas 164
31. Cooked Lentils 164
32. Homemade Applesauce 165

Conclusion **167**

Introduction

There is a good reason an anti-inflammatory diet is now one of the most talked-about diets, but before you can begin, you need to have a basic understanding of what inflammation is. Many individuals think that inflammation looks like puffy or reddish skin, as they get when they stub their toe. Inflammation may be seen in these two ways, but much more is happening.

Inflammation manifests itself because of the immune response that occurs inside the body. If your body is fighting an infection or has been damaged, it will send out cells that cause inflammation to help. This condition's symptoms might include swelling, redness, or occasional pain. Behavior that is natural and accepted in society.

If you can control your body—the story changes when the inflammation does not resolve itself and continues to be present. Chronic inflammation is linked to several diseases and conditions, including cardiovascular disease, Alzheimer's disease, type 2 diabetes, and cancer.

You are fortunate that you have some control over the degrees of inflammation. If you smoke cigarettes, are fat or overweight, or drink to excess (such as excessively), you may be more prone to inflammation. Altering one's diet, as opposed to using anti-inflammatory medication, may, so say some medical professionals, be an effective alternative to treating inflammation. It is also a good idea to limit the use of medication for chronic pain to just when it is necessary. This is because many drugs have undesirable side effects, such as drowsiness, confusion, and memory loss.

No official anti-inflammatory diet spells out precisely what, how frequently, and when one ought to eat certain foods and beverages. Consuming foods that have been shown to decrease inflammation and to avoid foods that have been shown to raise inflammation are two aspects of the anti-inflammatory diet. On the other hand, anti-inflammatory foods are meals that have been shown to reduce inflammation.

Brittany Scanniello, RD, an advocate for anti-inflammatory diets, suggests that rather than thinking of the meal as a diet, one should think of it as a way of life. She claims that eating anti-inflammatory foods "helps to minimize or control the low-grade inflammation that occurs throughout your body."

To maintain a healthy diet, it is essential to include a variety of plant-based foods such as fruits and vegetables, complex carbohydrates such as whole-grain bread and pasta, and a moderate quantity of dairy products and red meat.

Do you have an interest in learning more about anti-inflammatory foods and how they could assist you in preventing certain diseases? Onwards!

Chapter 1: Anti-inflammatory Diet - What to know?

Inflammation may act as a protective barrier for the body as a sign of illness to prevent additional harm. In most cases, it's an essential part of the healing process.

On the other hand, some people have a medical condition that makes their immune system less effective. This malfunction may lead to persistent or recurrent low-level inflammation.

Asthma, psoriasis, and rheumatoid arthritis are just a few conditions that may result in persistent inflammation. Evidence suggests that altering one's diet may help with the symptoms.

Fruits and vegetables, lean protein, whole grains, omega-3 fatty acids, healthy fats, and spices are all components of an anti-inflammatory diet. In this diet, processed foods, alcohol, and red meat are avoided or restricted.

A meal that reduces inflammation is more of an eating style than a diet. Meals that reduce inflammation include those that follow the DASH and Mediterranean diets.

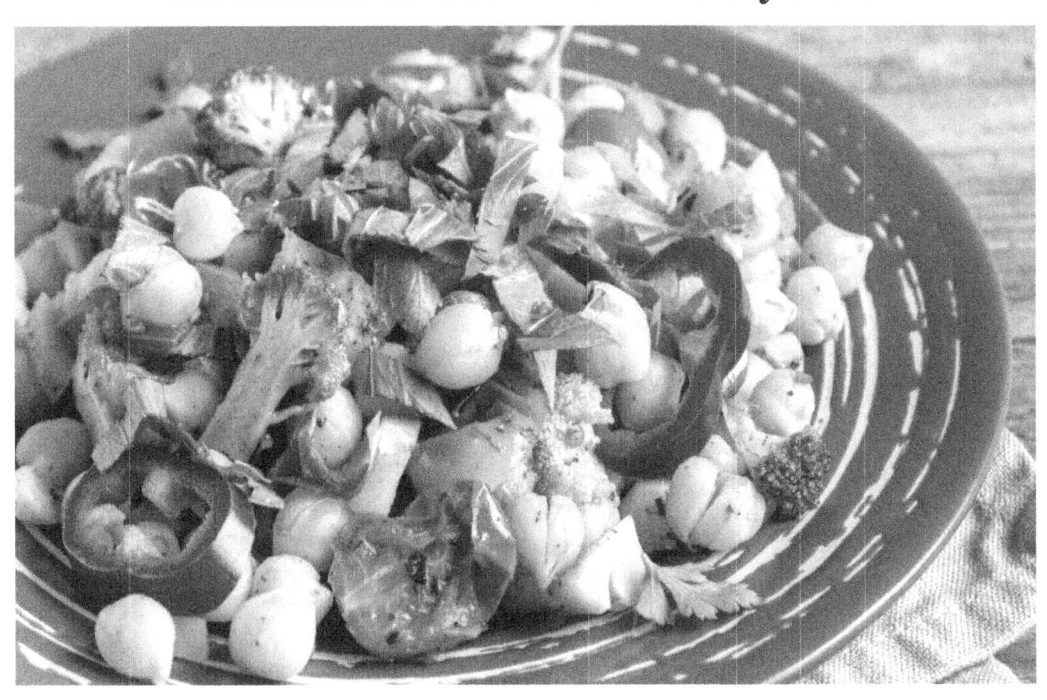

1.1 What is an anti-inflammatory diet?

A diet limited to processed foods is advised for patients with inflammatory illnesses. This recommendation includes beef.

Inflammation may be brought on or made worse by a few ingredients in food. Although complete, healthful foods are far less likely to have this effect, meals heavy in sugar and processed components may have it.

An anti-inflammatory lunch must include both fresh fruits and vegetables. Plant-based diets are rich in antioxidants. Conversely, certain foods may cause the body to produce radicals. Foods that are cooked in oil that has been heated repeatedly are one example.

Dietary antioxidants, substances in food, help the body eliminate free radicals. Free radicals are created by bodily processes like metabolism and then released into the environment. However, external factors like stress or cigarette use may raise the body's level of free radicals.

Free radicals may cause cell damage if they are present. Such damage has the potential to exacerbate or initiate several illnesses.

Although eating antioxidants are also helpful, the body naturally produces antioxidants that help it get rid of this toxic comb.

When leading an anti-inflammatory lifestyle, foods strong in antioxidants are recommended over those that increase levels of free radicals.

Omega-3 fatty acids, which are included in oily fish like salmon and tuna, may help reduce the body's synthesis of inflammatory mediators. The Arthritis Foundation claims that fiber could have a comparable effect.

1.2 Types of an anti-inflammatory diet

Many ketogenic diets already emphasize anti-inflammatory principles.

For example, the DASH and Mediterranean diets include heart-healthy fats, fresh fruits, vegetables, seafood, and whole grains.

A Mediterranean diet may lessen the harmful effects of inflammation on your cardiovascular system due to its concentration of plant-based foods and heart-healthy oils.

1.3 Who can it help?

Chronic inflammation is a factor in many illnesses and may be reduced by adopting anti-inflammatory habits.

One of the following conditions has inflammation:

- Psoriasis
- Asthma
- Rheumatoid arthritis
- Eosinophilic esophagitis
- Colitis
- Crohn's disease
- Inflammatory bowel diseases
- Hashimoto's thyroiditis
- Lupus
- Metabolic syndrome

A metabolic syndrome is a group of illnesses that includes type 2 diabetes, hypertension, obesity, and heart disease.

According to studies, each of these illnesses is influenced by inflammation. An anti-inflammatory lifestyle could be advantageous for those with metabolic syndrome.

Diets high in antioxidants may also help reduce the risk of several cancers.

1.4 Foods to eat

To combat inflammation, eat a diet rich in anti-inflammatory foods.

- Are abundant in nutrient
- Contain nourishing fats
- Provide a variety of antioxidants

Inflammation-fighting foods include:

- Oily fish, including salmon and tuna
- Fruits, including strawberries, blueberries, cherries, and blackberries
- Vegetables, including broccoli, kale, and spinach
- Fiber
- Beans

- Seeds and nuts
- Olive oil and olives
- moderately or raw, cooked veggies
- legumes, including lentils
- spices, including turmeric and ginger
- herbs
- prebiotics and probiotics
- tea

It's important to remember that no one meal can make someone's health better. It's crucial to eat a variety of healthy meals.

The best ingredients are created using just pure, natural substances. During processing, food may lose part of its nutritious content.

Consumers should carefully read the labels on prepared foods. However, even though cocoa is a fantastic alternative, it typically includes sugar and fat. A colorful dish may include many of the minerals and antioxidants in cocoa. You should incorporate colorful fruits and vegetables into your diet.

1.5 Foods to Avoid

People who are following an anti-inflammatory diet should avoid or eat the following as little as possible:

- processed foods
- foods including added salt or sugar
- unhealthful oils
- processed carbs that are present in white pasta, white bread, & a variety of baked goods
- processed snack meals, including crackers chips
- premade desserts, including ice cream cookies, and candy
- excess alcohol

People may also find it beneficial to decrease their consumption of the following:

Gluten: Some people get an inflammatory reaction after consuming gluten. A gluten-free diet has benefits and drawbacks, but it's not for everyone. It may be possible to reduce a person's symptoms by eliminating gluten for a while before deciding if it is beneficial.

Nightshades: Eating nightshade vegetables, including potatoes, peppers, tomatoes, and eggplants, may cause flare-ups in particular people with inflammatory diseases. There isn't much evidence to back up this assertion, but one might try cutting out nightshades from their diet for two to three weeks to see if their symptoms improve.

Carbohydrates: Several pieces of data indicate that a high-carb diet may cause inflammation in certain people even when the carbs are healthy for you. Despite high carbohydrate content, foods like sweet potatoes and whole grains are rich sources of antioxidants and nutrients.

1.6 Can a vegetarian diet reduce inflammation?

A vegetarian diet may be beneficial for those who desire to reduce inflammation. In 2019, the review's authors analyzed information from 40 studies. In the end, they discovered vegetarians had lower inflammatory marker levels than meat eaters.

In a study done in 2017 that looked at the dietary information of either Lacto-ovo vegetarians or non-vegetarians, there were 268 participants. The study's findings suggest that animal products may increase the risk of long-term inflammation and insulin resistance.

Research suggests that one significant benefit of a vegan diet may be lower levels of inflammation.

1.7 Anti-inflammatory diet tips

Adjusting a new diet may be challenging, but these tips might be helpful:

- When you go grocery shopping, choose a variety of fruits and vegetables as well as nutritious snacks.
- As you acclimate to them, replace fast meals with homemade lunches.
- You may use mineral water for soda and other calorie sweeteners.
- Asking your doctor about nutritional supplements, such as multivitamins or cod liver oil
- Schedule 30 minutes of moderate physical exercise every day.
- Practicing good sleep hygiene is essential since a lack of sleep may worsen inflammatory problems.

1.8 Takeaway

An anti-inflammatory diet may help treat symptoms of rheumatoid arthritis by reducing inflammation.

A diet high in fresh fruits, whole grains, veggies, and healthy fats may help manage inflammation, but no anti-inflammatory meal exists.

Anyone with a chronic illness that causes inflammation should discuss the best diet with their doctor.

1.9 11 Ways to Make the Most of An Anti-Inflammatory Diet + A Food List

Reducing inflammation could be helpful if you're attempting to eat healthfully over the long term. Chronic inflammation in the body exacerbates or worsens several debilitating chronic conditions, including rheumatoid arthritis, osteoarthritis, heart and brain disease, dementia, Alzheimer's disease, and Parkinson's disease.

Anti-inflammatory diets may help prevent certain diseases, but they may also help people age more slowly by controlling blood sugar levels and enhancing metabolism. Here are some of the most popular nutritional tips and recipes for meals that are low in inflammation.

1.10 Anti-inflammatory diet tips.

Follow these recommendations for an anti-inflammatory dinner for the most outstanding results:

25 g of fiber should be consumed each day.

When combined with a high-fiber diet, the natural anti-inflammatory phytonutrients found in fruits, vegetables, and whole foods may help reduce inflammation.

Vegetables, fruits, and whole grains are excellent sources of fiber. Excellent sources of fiber include whole grains like barley and oats, vegetables like okra and eggplant, fruits like bananas (3 g of fiber per banana), and blueberries (3.5 g of fiber per cup).

Aim for at least nine servings of fruit and vegetables each day.

One "serving" is half a cup of cooked fruits or vegetables or a cup of raw leafy vegetables.

Add turmeric, ginger, or other anti-inflammatory spices and herbs to increase their health benefits when cooking fruits and vegetables.

Eat four servings of crucifers and alliums per week.

Alliums and crucifers come in various varieties, but some popular ones include onions and garlic. Broccoli and cauliflower are examples of other cruciferous veggies.

Due to its high quantities of antioxidants, consuming an average of 4 servings each week may lower your chance of developing cancer. If you like the taste of garlic, it is advised to eat one clove daily.

You should consume 10% of your calories from saturated fat.

Reduce your intake of calories containing saturated fat to lower your risk of cardiovascular disease (approximately 20 g per 2,000 cal).

Red meat should only be consumed once a week and marinated with herbs, spices, and acidic raw fruit beverages to reduce the creation of dangerous compounds during cooking.

Consume a lot of omega-3-rich foods.

According to anecdotal evidence, omega-3 fatty acids have anti-inflammatory qualities and may lower the risk of chronic diseases, including cancer, heart disease, and arthritis.

To maximize your benefits, eat a variety of omega-3-rich foods, including walnuts, flax meal, and different beans like kidney, navy, and soy. It is also suggested to take a high-quality omega-3 supplement.

At the very least, try to consume fish three times a week.

A great source of omega-3 fatty acids is fish. Fish from cold water, such as salmon and oysters, are best. You might also choose trout, sardines, anchovies, herring, and mackerel.

Low-fat fish like sole and flounder may have anti-inflammatory qualities.

Replace low-fat oils with ones that are high in fat.

Although the body needs fat, you should only consume it if doing so would benefit your health.

Olive oils may have anti-inflammatory qualities (organic is preferred). Additional options include safflower, high-oleic, and expeller-pressed sunflower oil.

Two times every day, ideally in the middle of the day, have nutritious snacks.

Fruit, plain or unsweetened Greek-style yogurt, carrot and celery sticks, or nuts like almonds and pistachios are all terrific choices for a nutritious snack.

Avoid overly processed foods and sweets.

Your whole body becomes inflamed when you ingest meals high in salt or fructose syrup.

Avoid using refined sugars and artificial sweeteners at all costs. The dangers of consuming too much fructose include enhanced insulin sensitivity, raised uric acid and hypertension levels, and an increased risk of fatty liver disease.

Trans fats should be cut out of your diet completely.

According to studies, those who eat meals high in trans-fat have higher levels of protein C-reactive, a biomarker for inflammation. For this reason, the FDA mandated in 2006 that food manufacturers disclose trans fats on nutrition labels.

Generally, carefully read labels and steer clear of products marked "hydrogenated" or "half hydrogenated oils." Trans fatty acids are present in different levels in shortenings, crackers, margarine, and cookies.

Spices and fruit high in phytonutrients may be used to sweeten and flavor food.

Most fruits and vegetables are loaded with phytonutrients. Try including apricots, berries, apples, and even carrots to naturally sweeten your meals.

You may flavor savory recipes with anti-inflammatory spices as well. Cloves, cinnamon, thyme, turmeric, rosemary, and other anti-inflammatory herbs and spices are a few examples.

1.11 Best anti-inflammatory food list.

Just lately, there was a deluge of information about anti-inflammatory diets. To ensure you have everything you need in one place when you visit the grocery store, have a look at the following comprehensive list:

Vegetables

- onions
- eggplant
- okra
- scallions
- garlic
- carrots

- broccoli
- cabbage
- leek
- cauliflower
- Brussels sprouts
- mustard greens
- celery

Fruits

- blueberries
- apples
- bananas
- berries
- apricots

Whole grains

- oatmeal
- barley

Nuts, seeds, & legumes

- walnuts
- flax
- kidney beans
- navy beans
- almonds
- soybeans
- pistachios

Fish

- oysters

- herring
- salmon
- mackerel
- trout
- anchovies
- sardines

Herbs & spices

- ginger
- cloves
- turmeric
- cinnamon
- thyme
- Rosemary
- sage

1.12 Foods to avoid on an anti-inflammatory diet.

You should exclude foods and beverages that could be contributing to your body's inflammation in addition to consuming adequate anti-inflammatory meals. The following is a list of foods that you should avoid eating at all costs:

- Corn syrup High fructose
- Foods with High sodium
- Artificial sweeteners
- Refined sugar
- Partially Hydrogenated or hydrogenated oils

Incorporating more nutritious anti-inflammatory meals while reducing bad ones is the first step toward building a more substantial, healthier body.

1.13 61 Days Diet Plan

Day 1	
Breakfast	Quinoa Porridge with Chai-Infused Vanilla
Lunch	"Heart-Friendly" Salsa
Dinner	Portobello Mushroom Burgers

Day 2	
Breakfast	Power shake (alkaline avocado)
Lunch	Mushroom Risotto
Dinner	Magic Green Falafels

Day 3	
Breakfast	Quinoa bread
Lunch	Raw Energy Balls
Dinner	Roasted Tomato and Orange Soup Recipe

Day 4	
Breakfast	Basil overnight stone fruit oats
Lunch	Alkaline Wraps
Dinner	Green Detox Smoothie Bowl

Day 5	
Breakfast	Tropical Overnight Chia and Oats
Lunch	Avocado Couscous Salad Recipe
Dinner	Alkaline Lasagne

Day 6	
Breakfast	Chia Pudding with Layered Coconut Spirulina
Lunch	Chunky English Garden Salad Recipe
Dinner	Kale Detox Salad with Pesto

Day 7	
Breakfast	Detox Green Smoothie Monster
Lunch	Sunrise Turmeric Tonic
Dinner	Detox Rainbow roll-ups with peanut sauce

Day 8	
Breakfast	Detox Porridge with Whipped Berry
Lunch	Detox Wrap with Sunflower Seed Spread
Dinner	Comforting Cashew Curry

Day 9	
Breakfast	Acai Breakfast Bowl
Lunch	Spaghetti Squash Hash Browns
Dinner	Spicy Carrot & Greens

Day 10	
Breakfast	Kale Tapenade, Toast, and Avocado
Lunch	Roasted Vegetable Salad for Hormone Balance
Dinner	Roasted Cauliflower Detox Bowl

Day 11	
Breakfast	Grain, Nut & Gluten-Free Muesli
Lunch	Thai Cauliflower Rice Salad with Peanut Butter
Dinner	Easy Veggie Wrap with Avocado and Halloumi

Day 12	
Breakfast	Mango Mint Smoothie Bowl
Lunch	Tabbouleh
Dinner	Seven-Ved Stir-Fry 20

Day 13	
Breakfast	West Coast Avocado Toast
Lunch	Vegetable Stew
Dinner	Alkaline Cous-Cous

Day 14	
Breakfast	Chia Pudding
Lunch	Bliss Balls
Dinner	Thai Green Curry Made Alkaline

Day 15	
Breakfast	Fruit salad
Lunch	Raw Cacao Energy Balls
Dinner	Alkaline Wraps

Day 16	
Breakfast	Pecans with Roasted Pears
Lunch	Quinoa Bowl with Lentils and Mustard Vinaigrette
Dinner	Kale Slaw & Creamy Dressing

Day 17	
Breakfast	Berry Blast Porridge
Lunch	Perfectly Roasted Sweet Potato Fries
Dinner	Gaba Rice + A Mental-Health Supporting Bowl

Day 18	
Breakfast	Cycling Balls of Seed
Lunch	Split Pea Soup with Coconut (Spiced)
Dinner	Aubergine & Black Bean Alkaline Chili

Day 19	
Breakfast	Turmeric Tea with Golden Milk
Lunch	Miso-Harissa Delicate Squash and Brussels Sprouts Salad
Dinner	Stir-fry Mushroom and Broccoli

Day 20	
Breakfast	Beet Smoothie for Immune Strengthening
Lunch	One-Pot Curried Cauliflower with Couscous and Chickpeas
Dinner	Grilled Mackerel with Chili, Orange, Lemon, and watercress

Day 21	
Breakfast	Grapefruit and Blood Orange Salad with Cinnamon
Lunch	Grain Bowl with Spiced Squash & Mushrooms
Dinner	Quick Orecchiette Pasta with Kale Pesto

Day 22	
Breakfast	Chili Relleno Casserole
Lunch	Mediterranean Quinoa Salad with Roasted Veggies
Dinner	Vegetarian Pizza with Autumn Toppings

Day 23	
Breakfast	Breakfast Salad with Salsa Verde Vinaigrette
Lunch	Cinnamon Carrot Sticks
Dinner	Spicy Kimchi Tofu Stew

Day 24	
Breakfast	Breakfast Potatoes
Lunch	Foolproof Spinach & Feta Frittata
Dinner	Alkaline Chili Non-Carne
Day 25	
Breakfast	Camp Breakfast
Lunch	Lentil, Beetroot, and Hazelnut Salad
Dinner	Tomato Pie with Honey

Day 26	
Breakfast	Breakfast Strata
Lunch	Tofu Curry
Dinner	Black Bean Quinoa Burger with Activated Charcoal Bun

Day 27	
Breakfast	Superfood Breakfast
Lunch	Easy and Yummiest Kulfi Recipe
Dinner	Lentil Pasta with Kale and Marinara Sauce

Day 28	
Breakfast	Breakfast Pasta
Lunch	Guacamole
Dinner	Joseph's Best Easy Bacon Recipe

Day 29	
Breakfast	Breakfast Wellington
Lunch	Homemade Lunch Combination
Dinner	Alkaline Veggie Fajitas

Day 30	
Breakfast	Avocado & Kale Omelet
Lunch	Alkaline Wraps
Dinner	Aubergine & Chickpeas Balti

Day 31	
Breakfast	Transition Breakfast Muesli
Lunch	Tabbouleh
Dinner	Roasted Cauliflower, Fennel, and ginger Soup
Day 32	
Breakfast	Seedy Breakfast
Lunch	Bliss Balls
Dinner	Easy Kielbasa Skillet Dinner

Day 33	
Breakfast	Alkaline Fibre Muesli
Lunch	Vegetable Stew
Dinner	Easy Dinner Hash

Day 34	
Breakfast	Alkaline Baked Bean Salsa Brekkie
Lunch	Sunrise Turmeric Tonic
Dinner	Classic Carrot & Coriander Soup

Day 35	
Breakfast	Scrambled Tofu & Tomato Brekkie
Lunch	Tofu Curry
Dinner	Hobo Dinner

Day 36	
Breakfast	California Breakfast Salad
Lunch	Guacamole
Dinner	New Year's Day Dinner

Day 37	
Breakfast	Breakfast Potatoes
Lunch	Foolproof Spinach & Feta Frittata
Dinner	Alkaline Chili Non-Carne

Day 38	
Breakfast	Quinoa Porridge with Chai-Infused Vanilla
Lunch	"Heart-Friendly" Salsa
Dinner	Portobello Mushroom Burgers

Day 39	
Breakfast	Quinoa bread
Lunch	Raw Energy Balls
Dinner	Roasted Tomato and Orange Soup Recipe
Day 40	
Breakfast	Tropical Overnight Chia and Oats
Lunch	Avocado Couscous Salad Recipe
Dinner	Alkaline Lasagne

Day 41	
Breakfast	Detox Green Smoothie Monster
Lunch	Sunrise Turmeric Tonic
Dinner	Detox Rainbow roll-ups with peanut sauce

Day 42	
Breakfast	Acai Breakfast Bowl
Lunch	Spaghetti Squash Hash Browns
Dinner	Spicy Carrot & Greens

Day 43	
Breakfast	Grain, Nut & Gluten-Free Muesli
Lunch	Thai Cauliflower Rice Salad with Peanut Butter
Dinner	Easy Veggie Wrap with Avocado and Halloumi

Day 44	
Breakfast	West Coast Avocado Toast
Lunch	Vegetable Stew
Dinner	Alkaline Cous-Cous

Day 45	
Breakfast	Fruit salad
Lunch	Raw Cacao Energy Balls
Dinner	Alkaline Wraps

Day 46	
Breakfast	Superfood Breakfast
Lunch	Easy and Yummiest Kulfi Recipe
Dinner	Lentil Pasta with Kale and Marinara Sauce

Day 47	
Breakfast	Breakfast Wellington
Lunch	Homemade Lunch Combination
Dinner	Alkaline Veggie Fajitas

Day 48	
Breakfast	Power shake (alkaline avocado)
Lunch	Mushroom Risotto
Dinner	Magic Green Falafels

Day 49	
Breakfast	Basil overnight stone fruit oats
Lunch	Alkaline Wraps
Dinner	Green Detox Smoothie Bowl

Day 50	
Breakfast	Chia Pudding with Layered Coconut Spirulina
Lunch	Chunky English Garden Salad Recipe
Dinner	Kale Detox Salad with Pesto

Day 51	
Breakfast	Detox Porridge with Whipped Berry
Lunch	Detox Wrap with Sunflower Seed Spread
Dinner	Comforting Cashew Curry

Day 52	
Breakfast	Kale Tapenade, Toast, and Avocado
Lunch	Roasted Vegetable Salad for Hormone Balance
Dinner	Roasted Cauliflower Detox Bowl

Day 53	
Breakfast	Mango Mint Smoothie Bowl
Lunch	Tabbouleh
Dinner	Seven-Ved Stir-Fry 20

Day 54	
Breakfast	Chia Pudding
Lunch	Bliss Balls
Dinner	Thai Green Curry Made Alkaline

Day 55	
Breakfast	Pecans with Roasted Pears
Lunch	Quinoa Bowl with Lentils and Mustard Vinaigrette
Dinner	Kale Slaw & Creamy Dressing

Day 56	
Breakfast	Cycling Balls of Seed
Lunch	Split Pea Soup with Coconut (Spiced)
Dinner	Aubergine & Black Bean Alkaline Chili

Day 57	
Breakfast	Beet Smoothie for Immune Strengthening
Lunch	One-Pot Curried Cauliflower with Couscous and Chickpeas
Dinner	Grilled Mackerel with Chili, Orange, Lemon, and watercress

Day 58	
Breakfast	Chili Relleno Casserole
Lunch	Mediterranean Quinoa Salad with Roasted Veggies
Dinner	Vegetarian Pizza with Autumn Toppings

Day 59	
Breakfast	Breakfast Potatoes
Lunch	Foolproof Spinach & Feta Frittata
Dinner	Alkaline Chili Non-Carne
Day 60	
Breakfast	Breakfast Strata
Lunch	Tofu Curry
Dinner	Black Bean Quinoa Burger with Activated Charcoal Bun

Day 61	
Breakfast	Breakfast Pasta
Lunch	Guacamole
Dinner	Joseph's Best Easy Bacon Recipe

Chapter 2: Breakfast recipes

Breakfast is important in your daily diet. This chapter includes multiple types of alkaline breakfast recipes.

1. Quinoa Porridge with Chai-Infused Vanilla

Prep time: 5 mins, Cook time: 10 min, Servings: 2

Ingredients

- Dry quinoa 1 cup (organic)
- Water 2 cups (alkaline)
- Cinnamon 1 stick (or 1/2 tsp)
- Ground ginger 1 1/2 tsp/ finely grated fresh root ginger 1 "piece
- Ground nutmeg 1/2 tsp (fresh grated)
- Coconut cream 1/2 cup
- lemon skin grated 1/2 (or lime)
- Vanilla bean pod/vanilla essence 1
- Assorted nuts Sprinkle and seeds
- Cloves ground optional
- Grated apple 1 optional

Instructions

- As directed on the box, prepare the quinoa.
- The chai spices (ginger, cinnamon, nutmeg, and cloves if using a mortar and pestle), coconut milk, and vanilla bean should be added after the quinoa has been cooked and rinsed (add the vanilla essence, drop or 2)
- Depending on how thick and creamy you want, you may use either cream.
- When it's done, add the apple shreds before using them.

- Warm the meal before serving. Grate the lemon peel and top with cinnamon before serving (extra ground). Add the nuts and seeds last (sesame seeds are recommended).
- A tablespoon of coconut should be offered as a decadent choice. Its pH is alkaline.

Nutrition Facts Per Serving: Calories 516 | fat 19 g | Carbohydrate 55 g | Protein 12 g

2. Power shake (alkaline avocado)

Prep time: 15 mins, Cook time: 25 min, Servings: 2

Ingredients

- Cucumber 1
- Tomatoes 2
- Avocado 1
- Spinach leaves 1 handful
- Lime 1/2, juiced
- Red bell pepper ½ (a.k.a capsicum)
- Vegetable stock ½ tsp (organic & gluten-free)
- Warm water 50ml filtered

Optional

- Extra leaves (kale, lettuce, etc.)
- Herbs (parsley, basil, coriander)
- Spices (turmeric, ginger, cumin)

Instructions

- Before slicing the tomato, cucumber, bell pepper, and avocado finely, thoroughly wash each item.
- In 50 mL of warm water, dissolve the stock (vegetable).
- To produce a paste, combine the avocado and stock in a blender.
- Then, combine the products with a high-water content to make them more liquid.
- Vitamins, spinach, and lime should all be well blended.

- To serve, pour into a glass.
- If you have and prefer the optional components, add a few of them if you have them.

Nutrition Facts Per Serving: fat 18 g | Carbohydrate 40 g | Calories 317 | Protein 8 g

3. Quinoa bread

Prep time: 10 mins, Cook time: 20 min, Servings: 4

Ingredients

- Whole uncooked quinoa seed 300 g
- Water 1/2 cup
- Grapeseed oil 60 ml (¼ cup)
- Sea salt 1/2 tsp
- key lime 1/2, juiced

Instructions

- Quinoa should be refrigerated and soaked in water (overnight) (cold). Set the oven temperature to 320 degrees Fahrenheit (160 degrees Celsius).
- After draining the quinoa, rinse it in a sieve. Verify that the sieve has been cleared of any water. Quinoa and water should be combined in a food processor.
- In a mixing dish, combine key lime juice, grape seed oil, sea salt, and half a cup of water.
- Combine all ingredients in a food processor (3 mins). The bread batter will be uniform, with some quinoa still present.
- Spoon the batter pan with baking paper on the base and all four sides.
- Bake for 1.5 hours until the mixture is firm to the touch and gives slightly when finger pressure is applied.
- Allow it to cool in the pan for 30 minutes after taking it out of the oven. Cool on a rack after removing the cake from the pan. The bread will have a crispy crust and a moist inside.
- Let it completely cool before eating.

Nutrition Facts Per Serving: fat 13 g | Carbohydrate 5 g | Calories 152 | Protein 17 g

4. Basil overnight stone fruit oats

Prep time: 25 mins, Cook time: 35 min, Servings: 4

Ingredients

- Chia 2 tbsp
- Rolled oats ¾ cup
- Vanilla Silk Cashew Milk 1 cup
- Peach ½
- Plum ½
- basil leaves fresh 2 chopped roughly
- Pumpkin seeds 2 tsp
- Hemp seeds 2 tsp

Instructions

- Combine milk, oats, and chia seeds (Silk Vanilla Cashew). They need to be split across two serving dishes.
- To allow the oats to absorb the cashew milk, refrigerate overnight.
- Just before serving, toss with basil, fruit, and seeds.

Nutrition Facts Per Serving: fat 10 g | Carbohydrate 24 g | Calories 248 | Protein 13 g

5. Tropical Overnight Chia and Oats

Prep time: 25 mins, Cook time: 25 min, Servings: 5

Ingredients

- Chia 2 tbsp
- rolled oats 3/4 cup
- Silk Vanilla Cashew Milk 1 cup
- fresh mango cubed 1/4 cup
- Banana 1 (1/4 chopped)

- Avocado 1/2
- lemon juice 2 tsp

Instructions

- A good chia seed, oat, and milk mixture (Silk Vanilla Cashew). Two serving containers need to be made from them.
- Place the oats in the refrigerator overnight to help absorb the cashew milk.
- When prepared to serve, mix the whole banana, avocado, and lemon juice until they form a smooth puree. If required, add additional water to make a thicker puree.
- Toss the fruit purée, avocado, and chia-and-oat combination together.

Nutrition Facts Per Serving: fat 8 g | Carbohydrate 23 g | Calories 189 | Protein 4 g

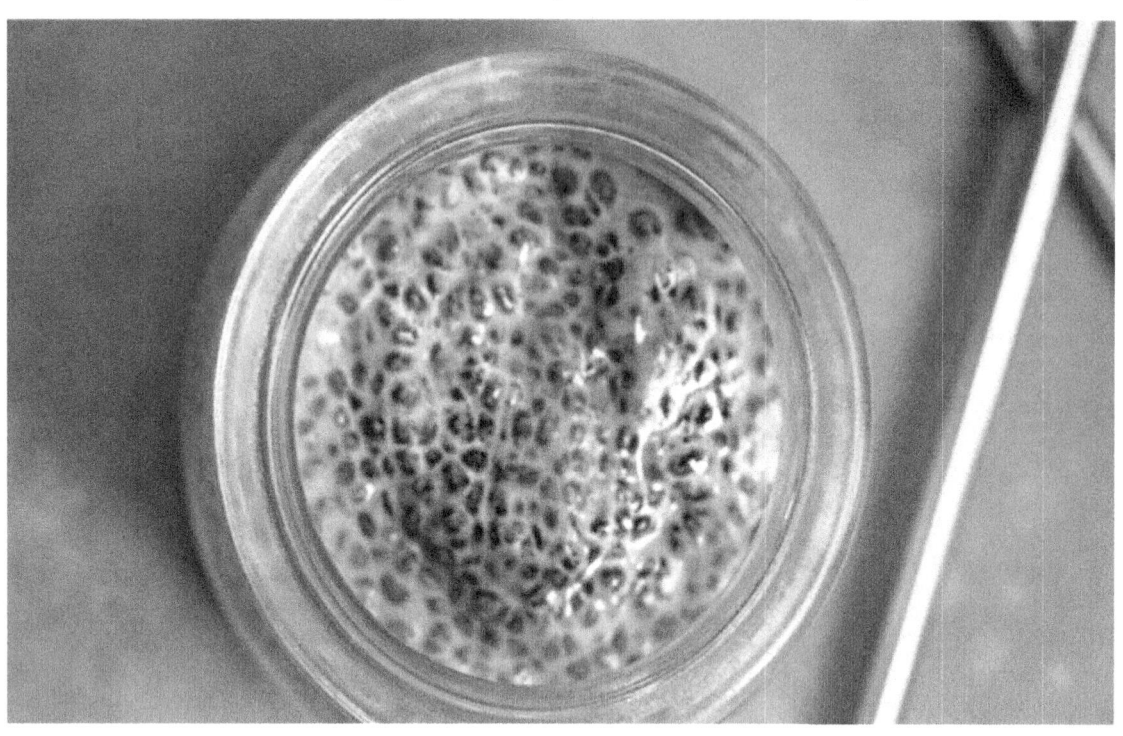

6. Chia Pudding with Layered Coconut Spirulina

Prep time: 5 mins, Cook time: 15 min, Servings: 2

Ingredients

- Chia seeds 5 tbsp.
- Almond milk 1 cup

- Organic coconut milk 1/2 cup
- Organic raw honey 2 tsp (replace it with agave/maple syrup if vegan)
- Avocado 1, peeled and cut into chunks
- Organic spirulina powder 1 tsp
- Banana 1 ripe, peeled
- For garnish: coconut flakes, fresh blueberries

Instructions

- Chia seeds, plant milk, and honey (or a replacement) should be combined in a medium dish. The mixture should be set aside for 30 minutes or until the seeds have absorbed the liquid.
- Meanwhile, blend the banana, avocado, and spirulina in a food processor until smooth.
- Spread the soaked chia evenly in the serving jars or bowls, top with a layer of spirulina puree to give it a green color, then top with chia seeds and coconut flakes to finish. Then, serve.

Nutrition Facts Per Serving: fat 13 g | Carbohydrate 5.6 g | Calories 125 | Protein 15 g

7. Detox Green Smoothie Monster

Prep time: 15 mins, Cook time: 15 min, Servings: 6

Ingredients

- Spinach (1 cup)
- Bee pollen (1 tbsp.)
- 1 apple (green & organic) cubes
- Spirulina powder (2 tsp)
- Banana (ripe) 1
- Almond milk (1/2 cup)
- lime juice (freshly squeezed) half cup
- One cucumber (cubes)

Instructions

- All components should be combined and blended well in a powerful blender.

Nutrition Facts Per Serving: fat 12 g | Carbohydrate 44 g | Calories 143 | Protein 9 g

8. Detox Porridge with Whipped Berry

Prep time: 5 mins, Cook time: 10 min, Servings: 5

Ingredients

- Rolled oats 1 cup
- Almond milk 1 cup
- 1 tsp
- Berries fresh/frozen 1 cup (I used blueberries)
- Organic raw honey 3 tsp
- Mixed seeds and sesame seeds, nuts chia, sunflower seeds, fresh mint leaves, hazelnuts, and 1 peach, sliced thinly, to garnish

Instructions

- Bring the milk and oats together in a small saucepan to a boil (medium heat).
- With frequent stirring, cook for 5 minutes.
- The berries, coconut oil, and honey should all be put in a blender and blended until smooth (smooth)
- Slices of peach, a mixture of seeds, and honey drizzled on top to taste are garnishes for serving.

Nutrition Facts Per Serving: fat 7 g | Carbohydrate 3 g | Calories 94 | Protein 6 g

9. Acai Breakfast Bowl

Prep time: 15 mins, Cook time: 10 min, Servings: 6

Ingredients

- Ripe bananas 2
- Acai powder 2 tbsp.
- Almond milk 1/2 cup
- Coconut oil 2 tsp
- Bee pollen 2 tsp
- Almond butter 1 tbsp.
- To garnish: crushed almonds, chia seeds, coconut flakes, acai berries, bee pollen,

Instructions

- Blend all ingredients and pulse to get a creamy mixture.
- Distribute evenly in serving bowls, then sprinkle with chia seeds, berries, pollen, and coconut flakes.

Nutrition Facts Per Serving: fat 8 g | Carbohydrate 6 g | Calories 112 | Protein 7 g

10. Kale Tapenade, Toast, and Avocado

Prep time: 20 mins, Cook time: 25 min, Servings: 8

Ingredients

- Free-range eggplants 2 poached
- Avocado 1 ripe peeled & cut into slices
- Tahini 2 tsp
- Pumpkin seeds 2 tsp
- Chia seeds 2 tsp
- Superfood tapenade 2 tbsp.
- Black pepper freshly ground

- Whole wheat good quality /gluten-free toast

For the tapenade

- Fresh kale leaves 1 cup
- Green pitted olives 1/2 cup
- Pumpkin seeds 1 tsp
- Spirulina 1/2 tsp
- Garlic clove 1
- Lemon juice 1 tbsp.
- Extra virgin olive oil 2 tsp
- Sea salt pinch

Instructions

On top of the tahini sauce, place slices of avocado.

Blend the ingredients for the tapenade twice, then transfer to a jar.

Spread a tablespoon. Toast should be topped with tapenade, chia seeds, and pumpkin before being served.

Nutrition Facts Per Serving: fat 11 g | Carbohydrate 5.4 g | Calories 189 | Protein 17 g

11. Grain, Nut & Gluten-Free Muesli

Prep time: 5 mins, Cook time: 25 min, Servings: 7

Ingredients

- Mixed seeds hemp, sunflower, chia, pumpkin, etc. 3 cups
- Mixed dried fruit apricot, apple, cranberry, etc. 1/2 cup
- Unsweetened coconut flakes 1/2 cup
- Fresh berries strawberry, raspberry, blueberry, etc. 1/2 cup
- Banana sliced 1
- Nondairy milk, almond, hemp, coconut, cashew, etc.

Instructions

- All dry ingredients should be combined and well mixed in a bowl. Take what you need for your bowl of cereal and put the other items in an airtight container—a foundation of sliced bananas. Add fresh berries and milk to the dry cereal.

Nutrition Facts Per Serving: fat 7 g | Carbohydrate 2 g | Calories 64 | Protein 5.4 g

12. Mango Mint Smoothie Bowl

Prep time: 5 mins, Cook time: 15 min, Servings: 4

Ingredients

- Mango (1 ripe), peeled & cut into chunks
- Almond butter (1 tbsp)
- Mint leaves approx. 5 to 6 (fresh)
- 1/2 cup low-fat coconut milk

Instructions

- All components should be combined and blended well in a powerful blender.

Nutrition Facts Per Serving: fat 14 g | Carbohydrate 9 g | Calories 364 | Protein 7.1 g

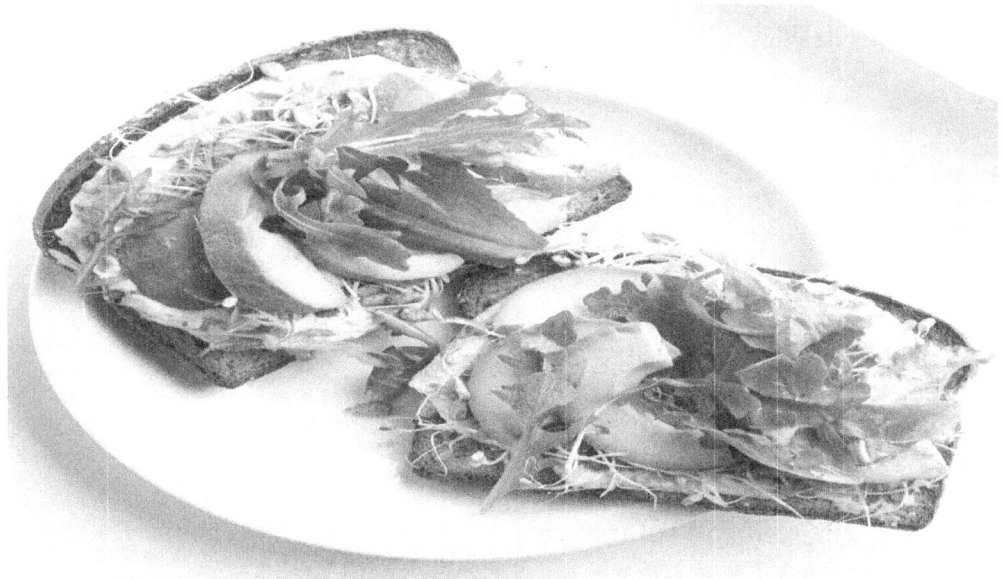

13. West Coast Avocado Toast

Prep Time: 10 Mins, Cook Time: 15 Mins, Serving: 1

Ingredients

- 1 cup salad greens mixed
- 1 tsp vinegar red wine
- 1 tsp olive oil extra-virgin
- salt Pinch
- pepper Pinch
- 2 slices of sprouted toasted whole-wheat bread
- ¼ cup plain hummus
- ¼ cup sprouts alfalfa
- ¼ sliced avocado
- 2 tsp sunflower seeds unsalted

Instructions

- Greens should be mixed with salt, vinegar, oil, and pepper, on every piece of bread and spread with hummus. On top, sprinkle sprouts, greens, avocado, and sunflower seeds.

Nutrition Facts Per Serving: fat 22 g | carbohydrate 46 g | calories 429 | protein 16 g

14. Chia Pudding

Prep time: 15 mins, Cook time: 30 min, Servings: 8

Ingredients

For the Chia Pudding

- almond milk 2/3 cup
- chia seeds 1/3 cup
- blueberries fresh 1/2 cup

For the Green Layer

- ripe avocado 1/2 peeled and cut into cubes
- spirulina powder 1/2 tsp

- fresh mint leaves 3-4
- bee pollen 1/2 tsp
- raw agave nectar 1 tsp
- almond milk 1/4 cup
- Fresh blueberries, mint leaves, and mixed nuts to garnish

Instructions

- Combine the blueberries, agave nectar, and almond milk in a blender to get a vibrantly colored liquid.
- Chia seeds should have 30 minutes to absorb all the liquid after being transferred to a plate, mixed in, and set away.
- Divide the pudding among the jars before serving.
- In a mixer, combine all the ingredients for the green smoothie and process until creamy.
- Distribute the mixture evenly among the serving jars after pouring it over the layer of chia pudding.
- Bee pollen and seeded mint leaves are used as a garnish. Packing may be done afterward.

Nutrition Facts Per Serving: fat 16 g | Carbohydrate 9 g | Calories 315 | Protein 32 g

15. Fruit salad

Prep time: 5 mins, Cook time: 15 min, Servings: 2

Ingredients

- Granulated sugar 75g
- Water 300ml
- 1 large lemon juice
- Cinnamon stick 1
- Pears 2 firm, peeled, cored & sliced
- Ripe peaches 2, peeled, stoned & chopped

- Pineapple rings 4 canned, drained & quartered
- Fresh raspberries 100g
- Blueberries 75g
- Redcurrants 75g, removed from stalks
- Ground mixed spice ½ tsp (optional)

Instruction

- The cinnamon stick, sugar, water, and lemon juice should be gently boiled until the sugar has completely dissolved. 3–4 minutes, or until syrupy, should be simmered. After turning off the heat, add the pear slices and place the pan aside to cool.
- Pour the cooled syrup and pears over the remaining fruit in a dish (remove the cinnamon stick). Gently stir for two hours, cover and chill. If you like, eat the fruit salad with a mixture of spices.

Nutrition Facts Per Serving: fat 18 g | Carbohydrate 14 g | Calories 402 | Protein 26 g

16. Pecans with roasted pears

Prep time: 10 mins, Cook time: 25 min, Servings: 6

Ingredients

- Pears 3
- Vanilla pods 2
- Butter 30g
- Pecans 50g

Instruction

- Set the oven's temperature to 200 C/400 F. Use a melon "baller" to scrape out all the seeds and sinewy bits of the core after cutting the pears half lengthwise.
- Cut the vanilla pods in half, then use a knife to scrape the seeds. Place the pears on a baking sheet, then divide the butter and vanilla seeds throughout the cavities of the pears. After 20 minutes of baking, sprinkle pecans on top and bake for 5 minutes.

Nutrition Facts Per Serving: fat 15 g | Carbohydrate 10 g | Calories 324 | Protein 21 g

17. Berry Blast Porridge

Prep time: 15 mins, Cook time: 15 min, Servings: 8

Ingredients

Porridge:

- Porridge oats 100g
- Milk/water 500ml
- Strawberries Handful quartered
- Raspberries Handful, whole

Redcurrant Compote:

- Redcurrants 100g
- Caster sugar 50g
- Orange juice 1 and zest

Instructions

- Redcurrant compote is made by removing the redcurrants and cooking sugar, orange juice, and zest in a small saucepan over low heat for 5 to 10 minutes or until the sugar has dissolved. Give it some time to cool.
- To create the porridge, mix the oats with the water (or milk if you want it creamier).
- Bring to a mild boil, then turn the heat down to low and simmer for 3 to 4 minutes, stirring occasionally.
- Place the strawberries and raspberries on top of the redcurrant compote that has been spooned over the porridge.

Nutrition Facts Per Serving: fat 26 g | Carbohydrate 5 g | Calories 299 | Protein 16 g

18. Cycling Balls of Seed

Prep time: 15 mins, Cook time: 25 min, Servings: 6

Ingredients

- Raw pumpkin seeds 7 tbsp.
- Flaxseed 7 tbsp.
- Almond butter 1 tbsp.
- Pitted dates soaked 4 dry and drained
- Coconut oil 1 tbsp.
- Rolled oats 2 tbsp.
- Matcha powder 1 tbsp. plus extra for coating
- Almond milk 1 tbsp.

Instructions

- To produce flour, pulse the peas, flax, and pumpkin seeds in a food processor.
- The remaining ingredients should be processed until a sticky mixture forms. Add more milk if the mixture is too dry (almond).
- Form the mixture with your hands, then set the balls on a matcha powder plate.
- Before transferring to an airtight glass jar and chilling for at least an hour before serving, roll to coat evenly.
- Maintain in the fridge for up to a week.

Nutrition Facts Per Serving: fat 17 g | Carbohydrate 12 g | Calories 367 | Protein 14 g

19. Turmeric Tea with Golden Milk

Prep time: 10 mins, Cook time: 15 min, Servings: 3

Ingredients

- Unsweetened non-dairy milk 1 cup, preferably coconut milk
- Cinnamon stick 1 (3")

- Turmeric 1 (1") piece, unpeeled, sliced thinly / dried turmeric 1/2 tsp
- Ginger 1 (1/2") piece, unpeeled, sliced thinly
- Honey 1 tbsp.
- Virgin coconut oil 1 tbsp.
- Whole black peppercorns 1/4 tsp
- For serving Ground cinnamon

Instructions

- Mix the cinnamon, coconut milk, turmeric, ginger, sugar, peppercorns, and 1 cup of water in a saucepan. Then, slowly bring it to a low boil—Cook for 10 minutes, or until the flavors have melted, over low heat. Pour into cups using a fine-mesh filter, then sprinkle some cinnamon.

Nutrition Facts Per Serving: fat 22.5 g | Carbohydrate 11.5 g | Calories 402 | Protein 29 g

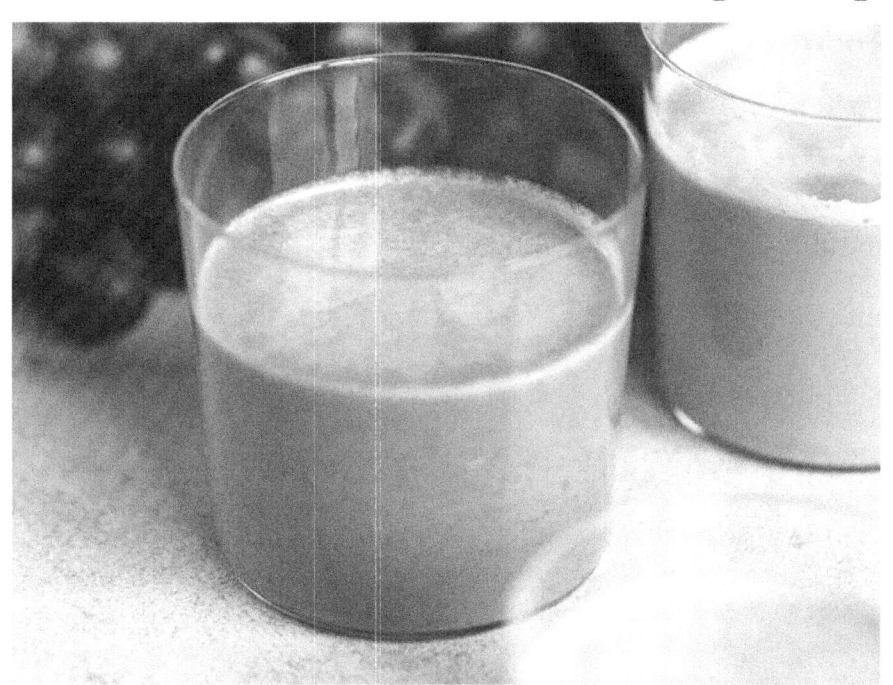

20. Beet Smoothie for Immune Strengthening

Prep time: 5 mins, Cook time: 15 min, Servings: 6

Ingredients

- Beet peeled med 1 and cut into small cubes

- Raspberries fresh/frozen 1 cup
- Grapefruit 1 peeled & cut into slices
- Lemon juice freshly squeezed 1 tbsp.
- Chia seeds 2 tsp
- Unsweetened almond milk 1/2 cup
- Ginger piece ½" peeled and grated

Instructions

- Combine the ingredients in a blender.
- Blend the drink until it's creamy and smooth.
- To make beautiful layers, split the mixture into glasses once you've poured the smoothie.
- Use a spoon toss before serving.

Nutrition Facts Per Serving: fat 8 g | Carbohydrate 34 g | Calories 342 | Protein 17 g

21. Grapefruit and Blood Orange Salad with Cinnamon

Prep time: 5 mins, Cook time: 10 min, Servings: 5

Ingredients

- Pink grapefruits 2 large
- Blood oranges 2
- Extra-virgin olive oil 1/4 cup
- Raw apple cider vinegar 2 tbsp.
- Sea salt 1/2 tsp
- Chopped fresh sage 1/4 cup
- Black pepper freshly ground
- Ground cinnamon 1/2 tsp, for dusting

Instructions

- Start by leaving the fruit's skins on to make slicing them into small slices simpler. Slice the oranges and grapefruits into little circles using a knife. The shell of each circular frame should be taken off. You may do it with your thumbnail or by making a little cut in the peel and beginning to cut it off. To protect the spherical frame throughout this procedure, you should use caution.

- Mix the olive oil, mustard, salt, sage, and pepper to taste in a small bowl.

- Arrange the fruit rounds in contrasting colors on a large tray or dish. Toss with the vinaigrette and cinnamon just before serving. Refrigerate in an airtight glass jar or serve immediately (1 day).

Nutrition Facts Per Serving: fat 12.8 g | Carbohydrate 28.4 g | Calories 403 | Protein 23.1 g

22. Chili Relleno Casserole

Prep Time: 10 Mins, Cook Time: 35 Mins, Serving: 8

Ingredients:

- 3 eggplants
- ¾ cup half-n-half
- What you'll need from the store cupboard:
- 2 (7 oz.) cans of whole green chilies, drain well
- ½ tsp salt
- Nonstick cooking spray

Instructions:

- The oven temperature is set at 350. Cooking spray should be used to coat an 8-inch baking pan.
- Each chili is flattened after being cut along its long side. Place half of the chili's skin side down in a single layer in the baking pan that has been prepared.
- Add the pepper and the remaining chilies, skin side up, on top.
- Beat the eggplants, salt, and half-and-half in a small bowl. Pour over the peppers.
- Bake for 35 minutes or until golden brown on top. 10 minutes should pass before serving.

Nutrition Facts Per Serving: fat 13 g | carbohydrate 36 g | calories 295 | protein 13 g

23. Breakfast Salad with Salsa Verde Vinaigrette

Prep Time: 10 Mins, Cook Time: 10 Mins, Serving: 1

Ingredients

- 3 tbsp Verde salsa
- 1 tbsp extra-virgin divided olive oil
- 2 tbsp chopped cilantro
- 2 cups of mesclun
- 8 tortilla chips, blue corn
- ½ cup of canned red rinsed kidney beans
- ¼ sliced avocado

Instructions

- In a mixing dish, combine the cilantro, 1 tbsp of oil, and salsa. Mesclun and half of the mixture should be combined on a small plate.
- Add avocado, beans, and chips as a salad topping.
- A compact nonstick skillet. Over a moderate burner, warm the oil.
- Serve the mixture besides the salad. Add more cilantro as a garnish if desired, and then dress the salad with the remaining salsa vinaigrette.

Nutrition Facts Per Serving: fat 34 g | carbohydrate 37 g | calories 527 | protein 16 g

24. Breakfast Potatoes

Prep Time: 20 Mins, Cook Time: 30 Mins, Serving: 4

Ingredients

- 4 medium russet potatoes
- 1 onion, chopped
- 2 tbsp olive oil
- 1 tbsp ground cumin

- 1 pinch salt and ground black pepper to taste
- ¼ cup butter, cut into 4 pieces
- 4 slices bacon, chopped

Instructions

- Prepare the dish and preheat the oven to 350 degrees Fahrenheit (175 deg C).
- In a mixing bowl, combine the potatoes and onion. Cut into fourths. Add the cumin, oil, salt, pepper, and olive oil as desired. The dish should be covered with plastic wrap before baking.
- On the baking sheet, distribute the potato-onion mixture evenly. One slice of butter should be placed on top of each potato corner.
- The potatoes should be fork soft after baking in a preheated oven for 30 minutes.
- While the potatoes bake, cook the bacon for 10 to 12 minutes over medium heat, often tossing. Drain on a platter covered with paper towels.
- Place the hot, freshly baked potatoes on a serving plate. Add the bacon and Cheddar to taste.

Nutrition Facts Per Serving: fat 13 g | Carbohydrate 44 g | Calories 415 | Protein 11 g

25. Camp Breakfast

Prep Time: 15 mins, Cook Time: 26 mins, Serving: 2

Ingredients

- 6 slices cut crosswise bacon
- 1 tbsp of olive oil
- 3 cubed white potatoes
- to taste, salt & black pepper ground
- 1 chopped onion
- 4 beaten eggplants

Instructions

- Over medium heat, cook and stir the bacon for 5 minutes or until crispy. Most of the oil should be discarded after transferring to a plate covered with paper towels to drain.

- Over medium heat, warm the olive oil in a skillet. Stir regularly and cook the potatoes for approximately 10 minutes or until they are crispy and golden.

- Toss the potatoes and onion together and cook for 5 minutes until the onion is transparent. To ensure the bacon is well cooked, heat for 1–2 minutes while tossing often.

- The eggplants should be cooked and whisked over the potato mixture for 5–6 minutes or until they are set.

Nutrition Facts Per Serving: fat 19 g | Carbohydrate 49 g | Calories 362 | Protein 28 g

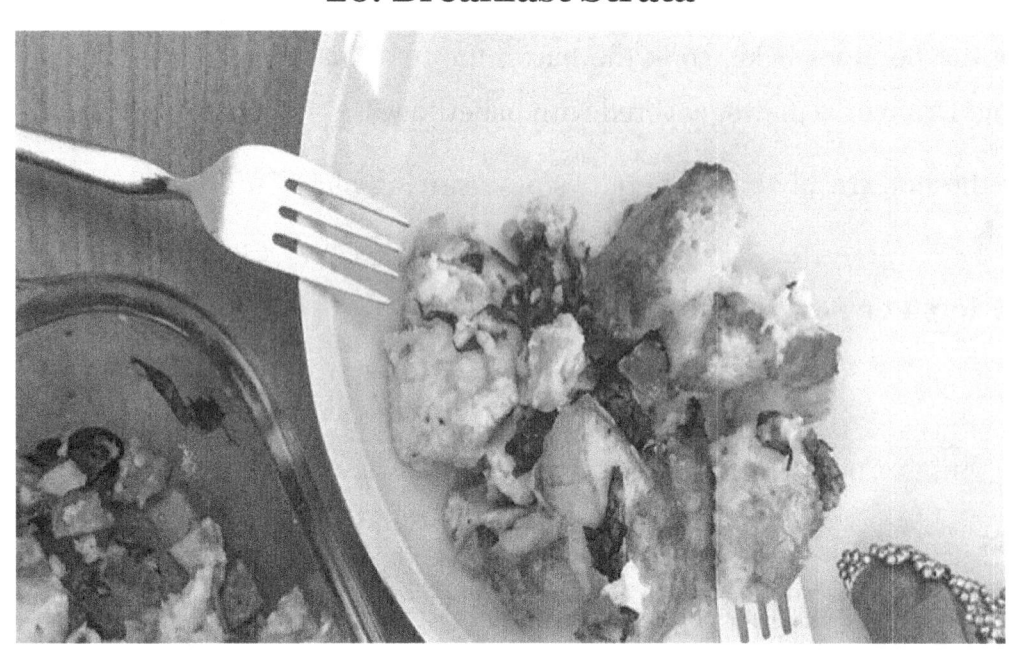

26. Breakfast Strata

Prep Time: 20 mins, Cook Time: 1 hr 15 mins, Serving: 8

Ingredients

- 1 lb casings removed from the sausage
- 2 cups fresh mushrooms sliced
- 10 cups of day-old bread cubed
- 3 cups whole milk

- 1 & ½ cups Forest ham cubed Black
- 1 package frozen thawed & drained, chopped spinach
- 2 tbsp flour all-purpose
- 2 tbsp powdered mustard
- 1 tsp salt
- 3 tsp melted butter
- 2 tsp basil dried

Instructions

- Oil a 9 by 13-inch casserole dish very lightly.
- Sausage should be cooked and stirred for about 10 minutes or until crumbled and well-browned. Place the cooked sausage in the casserole dish that has been set aside.
- Cook and stir mushrooms in a skillet over medium heat for 5–10 minutes, or until liquid is released and they are lightly browned; drain.
- Except for the sausage, combine all the ingredients in a large mixing basin and toss well. After that, add the mixture on top. Place the casserole dish in the refrigerator overnight or for at least two hours.
- Turn the oven temperature to 350 degrees (175 deg C).
- Bake in a preheated oven for 60 to 70 minutes or until a knife inserted in the middle comes out clean.

Nutrition Facts Per Serving: fat 17 g | Carbohydrate 32 g | Calories 400 | Protein 23 g

27. Superfood Breakfast

Cook time: 5 mins, Prep Time: 5 mins, Serving: 1

Ingredients

- ¼ cup of blueberries
- 2 tbsp goji berries dried
- 1 tbsp flax seed ground

- 1 tbsp walnuts ground
- 1 tbsp almonds ground
- 1 tsp cocoa powder unsweetened
- ½ tsp cinnamon ground
- ½ tsp of honey

Instructions

- In a dish, combine the goji berries, blueberries, & flaxseed to make the granola.

Nutrition Facts Per Serving: fat 11 g | Carbohydrate 43 g | Calories 347 | Protein 20 g

28. Breakfast Pasta

Prep time: 10 mins, cook time: 30 mins, Serving: 4

Ingredients

- ½ package of spaghetti
- 3 tbsp divided olive oil
- 4 beaten eggplants
- ½ diced onion
- ¼ cup baby Bella mushrooms chopped
- ¼ cup frozen peas
- ¼ cup shredded carrots
- salt & black pepper ground

Instructions

- With a pinch of salt, bring a big pot of water to a boil. In a big pot of boiling water, cook the spaghetti for 12 minutes or until it's al dente but still firm to the biting. Drain.
- For approximately 5 minutes, cook and whisk the eggplants in the heated oil until they are firm and scrambled. Oil should be heated in a medium-sized pan.
- For approximately 10 minutes, or until the onion is golden, sauté the mushrooms, peas, onion, and carrots in a separate skillet of heated oil over medium-high heat. In a large

mixing basin, combine the spaghetti and the onion mixture. The eggplants should be thoroughly combined in a large mixing dish. Toss the freshly grated Parmesan, salt, and pepper with the spaghetti mixture.

Nutrition Facts Per Serving: fat 17 g | Carbohydrate 42 g | Calories 412 | Protein 18 g

29. Breakfast Wellington

Prep Time: 15 mins, Cook Time: 45 mins, Serving: 12

Ingredients

- 1 lb sausage ground
- 1 package thawed broccoli chopped frozen
- ½ cup cream sour
- 2 cans rolled refrigerated dough crescent

Instructions

- Set the oven temperature to 325 degrees Fahrenheit (165 deg C).
- In a big, shallow pan, brown sausage on both sides for about 10 minutes. Cook until both sides are uniformly browned over medium heat. Drain, crush, and store in a different container for later use.
- Frozen broccoli should be heated in a covered pan for 5 minutes over medium heat.
- Add all ingredients to a large mixing basin and combine well.
- One crescent roll packet should be flattened and placed in a baking dish. Add the broccoli mixture on top. Using a serrated knife, seal the remaining crescent rolls around the filling.
- In a preheated oven, bake for 20 minutes or until golden brown.

Nutrition Facts Per Serving: fat 21 g | Carbohydrate 27 g | Calories 326 | Protein 11 g

30. Avocado & Kale Omelet

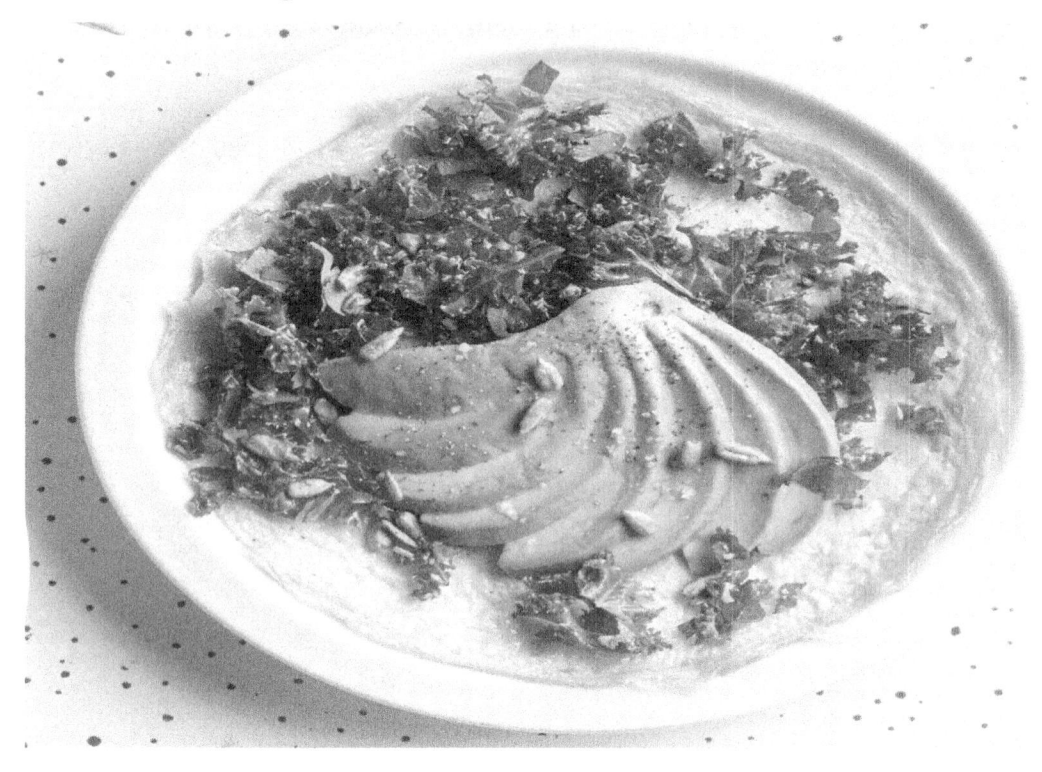

Prep Time: 10 Mins, Cook Time: 10 Mins, Serving: 1

Ingredients

- 2 eggplants large
- 1 tsp milk low-fat
- salt Pinch
- 2 tsp of extra-virgin divided olive oil
- 1 cup chopped kale
- 1 tbsp lime juice
- 1 tbsp fresh cilantro chopped
- 1 tsp sunflower seeds unsalted
- red pepper crushed Pinch
- salt Pinch
- ¼ sliced avocado

Instructions

- It would be best if you had a small bowl to quickly prepare a batch of beaten eggplants with fresh milk and salt. Put a nonstick pan over medium-high heat and add 1 teaspoon of oil. Cook for another minute or two if the center is still a bit runny, but the base has set. Turn it over when it is set on the second side and continue heating it for thirty seconds or until it is well cooked. Transfer to a serving plate after that to cool.
- Add sunflower seeds, chopped cilantro, and a dash of salt as a garnish. Before serving, add avocado and kale salad to the omelet.

Nutrition Facts Per Serving: fat 28 g | carbohydrate 9 g | calories 339 | protein 15 g

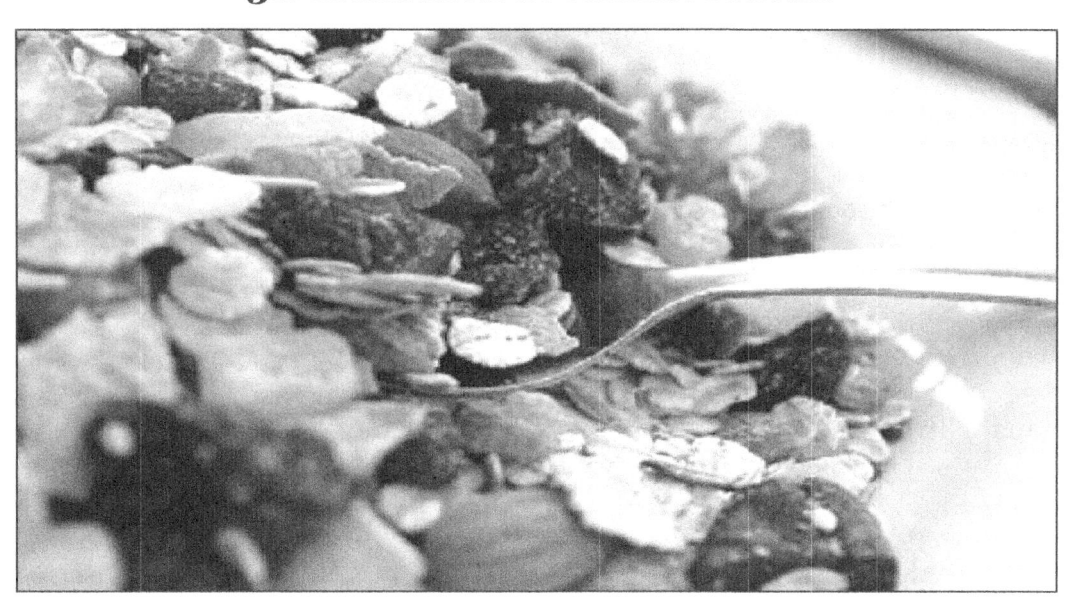

31. Transition Breakfast Muesli

Prep time: 5 mins, Cook time: 0 min, Servings: 2

Ingredients

- Organic oats
- Handful almonds
- Handful walnuts
- Handful cranberries
- 1 banana
- Rice milk for taste

Instructions

- Combine the ingredients, then serve with your preferred milk.

Nutrition Facts Per Serving: Calories 435|fat 18 g | Carbohydrate 51 g| Protein 23 g

---

32. Alkaline Fibre Muesli

Prep time: 5 mins, Cook time: 0 min, Servings: 2

Ingredients

- Toasted oats
- A handful of almond meal
- A small handful of psyllium husks
- Sliced almonds
- Sunflower seeds, sliced
- Handful of buckwheat
- 1/2 apple, grated
- cinnamon & nutmeg
- Almond milk for taste

Instructions

- Mix all ingredients and as much milk as you want to create muesli.

Nutrition Facts Per Serving: Calories 419|fat 9 g | Carbohydrate 45 g| Protein 22 g

---

33. Seedy Breakfast

Prep time: 5 mins, Cook time: 0 min, Servings: 2

Ingredients

- 2 cups sunflower seeds with 2 cups pumpkin seed
- 2 cups almonds
- 2 cups sesame seeds with 1 apple, grated
- Alkaline water

- soy milk, 25ml

Instructions

- For three hours, the seed and apple mixture should be soaked in soy milk and alkaline water.
- To change the flavor, you can add more soy milk when it's finished.

Nutrition Facts Per Serving: Calories 399|fat 12 g | Carbohydrate 48 g| Protein 22 g

34. Alkaline Bean Salsa Baked Brekkie

Prep time: 30 mins, Cook time: 0 min, Servings: 2

Ingredient

- 1 can haricot beans
- 6 cherry tomatoe
- 4 spring onions
- 2 handfuls spinach
- 2 cloves garlic
- 1 avocado
- ½ Olive oil, lemon
- 1 handful basil
- Himalayan salt with black pepper

Instructions

- Slice the cherry tomatoes in half, the garlic thinly, and all the spring onions coarsely. In a medium-sized frying pan with around 50 ml of water, "steam fried" the garlic for a minute.
- Currently, add beans, cherry tomatoes, and haricot spring onions. It shouldn't take more than a minute to do this.
- At this stage, add the basil and spinach and simmer until just wilted. Then, season with black pepper and Himalayan salt.
- Once the avocado has been cut in half while cooking, everything is ready.

- The bean salsa mixture may be served with a salad and a half avocado drizzled with olive oil and lemon.

Nutrition Facts Per Serving: Calories 413|fat 8 g | Carbohydrate 42 g| Protein 19 g

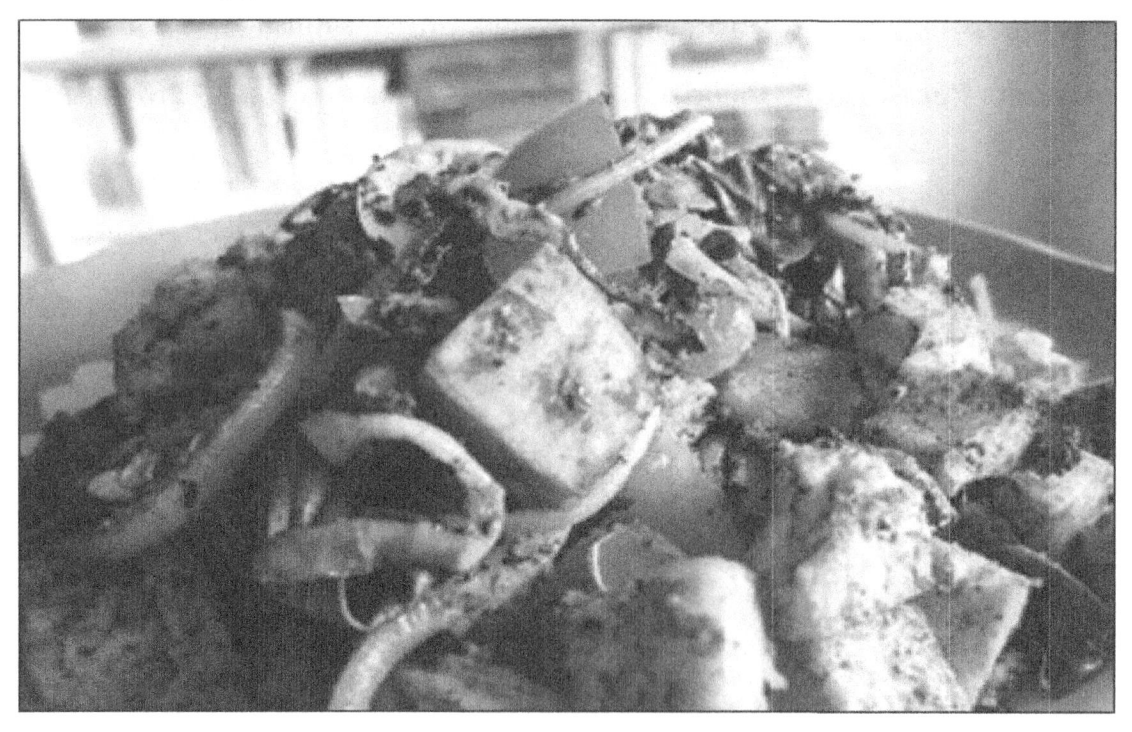

35. scrambled Tofu & Tomato Brekkie

Prep time: 15 mins, Cook time: 0 min, Servings: 2

Ingredients

- firm tofu, 285g
- 1 tbsp. of coconut oil
- 2 tomatoes
- ½ brown onion
- ½ red pepper
- Turmeric pinch
- Black pepper
- Sea salt
- 1little basil

Instructions

- You can finish this in a few minutes. Tofu may be added to the mixture by chopping or crumbling it with your hands in a bowl. Cut the onion and pepper, and quickly fry them in coconut oil.

- Tofu, chopped tomatoes, and a dash of turmeric should all be combined in a pan. While the tofu cooks, add the salt and black pepper by grinding them. Add a couple of basil leaves at the end, and you're done!

- It tastes best when topped with some baby spinach leaves, olive oil, and toasted sprouted bread.

Nutrition Facts Per Serving: Calories 441|fat 12.5 g | Carbohydrate 49 g| Protein 9 g

36. California Breakfast Salad

Prep Time: 10 Mins, Cook Time: 03 Mins, Serving: 1

Ingredients

- 1 large egg(s)
- 2 tsp Balsamic Vinegar White
- 2 tsp olive oil extra-virgin
- 1 & ½ cups Mix Baby Lettuce
- 4 leaf basil leaves fresh
- ½ cup Tomatoes Grape
- ¼ cup red onion
- 1/3 avocado medium
- 1/8 tsp salt sea
- ¼ tsp black pepper ground

Instructions

- Cooking spray should be heated to a hot but not smoking temperature on a small nonstick skillet (without PFOA). Then, cook it to your desired doneness.

- Meanwhile, mix the vinegar and oil in a serving dish. Olive oil and salt, and pepper should be sprinkled on before serving.
- The salad should be served with cooked eggplant seasoned with salt and pepper.

Nutrition Facts Per Serving: fat 21 g | carbohydrate 20 g | calories 213| protein 10 g

Chapter 3: Lunch Recipes

In your busy schedule a healthy and delicious lunch will make you active for your work. Here you will find diverse alkaline and anti-inflammatory lunch recipes.

1. "Heart-Friendly" Salsa

Prep time: 25 mins, Cook time: 35 min, Servings: 4

Ingredients

- Blueberries 1 Cup
- Strawberries 5
- Sea Salt 1 Pinch
- Grape Seed Oil 2 Tbsp.
- Red Onion 1/4
- Green Bell Pepper Chopped 1/3 Cup
- Chopped Avocado 1/2
- Two Key Limes Juice

Instructions

- Blueberries, key lime juice, onion, key lime zest, strawberries, and green bell pepper should all be added to a food processor or blender and pulsed about 5 to 6 times.
- Add sea salt and cayenne pepper for flavoring, if preferred.
- In a mixing basin, scrape the salsa and include the diced avocado.

Nutrition Facts Per Serving: fat 18.7 g | Carbohydrate 38 g | Calories 359 | Protein 27.2 g

2. Mushroom Risotto

Prep time: 15 mins, Cook time: 35 min, Servings: 2

Ingredients

- Grapeseed Oil 1 Tbsp.
- Mushrooms 4
- Sea Salt
- Cayenne Pepper
- Onion 1/2
- Wild Rice 2 Cups
- Homemade Vegetable Broth 4 Cups

Instructions

- On medium heat, sauté the mushrooms and onions in grapeseed oil. Cook, often stirring, for 5 to 7 minutes or until the mushrooms are finely browned, and the liquid has evaporated.
- Add the rice and boil for an additional minute.
- Apply the extra sea salt, black pepper, and broth to the vegetables. For approximately two hours, cover and simmer. Likewise, cook the rice for 45 minutes at low heat or 1 hour and 15 minutes at high heat or until soft.

Nutrition Facts Per Serving: fat 8 g | Carbohydrate 29.4 g | Calories 289 | Protein 12 g

3. Raw Energy Balls

Prep time: 15 mins, Cook time: 25 min, Servings: 6

Ingredients

- Blueberries 1/2 Cup
- Shredded Coconut 2 Cups
- Walnuts 1/2 Cup
- Dried Dates 1/2 Cup

- Date Sugar 1 Tsp.
- Agave Syrup 1 Tbsp.
- Sea Salt 1 Pinch

Instructions

- First, pulse the walnuts or Brazil nuts in a powerful blender or food processor to make the powder.
- Mix the blueberries, dry dates, and date sugar in a bowl. The agave syrup should be drizzled in gradually until you have a paste.
- For up to two hours, refrigerate the mixture.
- Roll them in additional coconut, if desired, after shaping them into 1 tbsp balls. In the refrigerator, it will keep for about a week and it three months in the freezer.

Nutrition Facts Per Serving: fat 8 g | Carbohydrate 38.4 g | Calories 356 | Protein 19 g

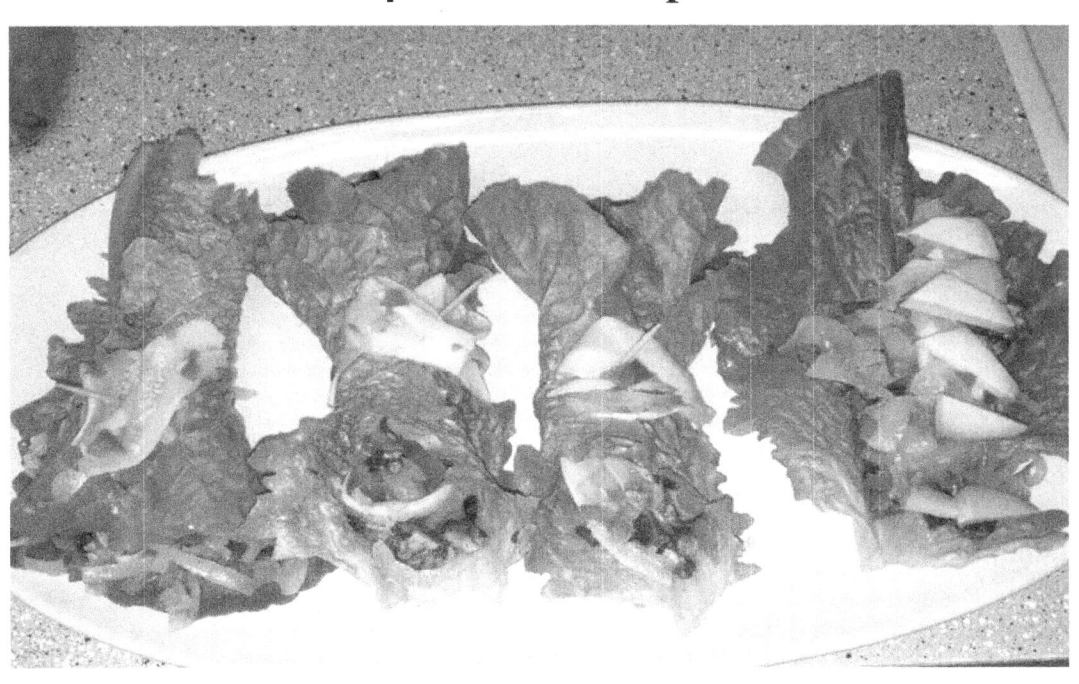

4. Alkaline Wraps

Prep time: 20 mins, Cook time: 0 mins, Servings: 2

Ingredients:

- 6 large leaves of romaine lettuce

- 2 ripe tomatoes
- 3 ripe avocados
- ½ red onion
- ½ chili
- 1/2 bunch of coriander
- Juice of one organic lemon
- 1 pinch of sea salt

Instructions

- Mash your avocados first. Before incorporating the tomatoes and other ingredients, crush or dice them. Next, season the avocado with salt and lemon juice, and combine it with the chopped ingredients. It resembles salsa but contains a lot more avocados. The pH balance in the alkaline range is ideal.
- Wash and pat dry the large lettuce leaves first.
- The mixture should be wrapped in leaves and secured with a cocktail stick.

Nutrition Facts Per Serving: Calories 379 | fat 11 g | Carbohydrates 38 g | Protein 29 g

5. Avocado Couscous Salad Recipe

Prep time: 20 mins, Cook time: 30 min, Servings: 6

Ingredients

- Avocados 2
- Couscous 500g
- Lemon juice 1tbsp
- drained chickpeas 1 x 220g
- Red pepper 1
- Pomegranate 1
- Orange juice 4tbsp

- Virgin olive oil 2tbsp
- Chopped mint 2tbsp
- Flat-leaf parsley 1tbsp
- toasted pine nuts 100g

Instructions

- Add boiling water to the couscous and cover. Wrap in a tea towel, then soak for 20 minutes (damp). Use a fork to break up the grains.
- Before cutting the avocado into slices, peel, and stone it. The mixture with the lemon juice.
- Toss the couscous with the avocado, chickpeas, and pepper you've combined in a bowl.
- To get the seeds out, cut the pomegranate in half. Do it over a plate so you can collect any liquids. Sprinkle the seeds over the couscous.
- Add the oil and the juices of the orange and lemon. Fork through after tossing the couscous with the herbs and dressing. Pine nuts should be sprinkled on top before serving.

Nutrition Facts Per Serving: fat 14.6 g | Carbohydrate 37.3 g | Calories 369 | Protein 21 g

6. Chunky English Garden Salad Recipe

Prep time: 20 mins, Cook time: 25 min, Servings: 2

Ingredients

- Cucumber 1
- Lettuces 2 small
- Radishes 8
- Mint leaves as per your taste
- Lemon juice
- Olive oil
- Black pepper and Sea salt

Instructions

- After slicing the cucumber into four or six slices, cut each slice into a wedge.

- Place the cucumber, radish, torn mint leaves, and each lettuce leaf cut into thirds on a serving platter.
- On top, drizzle copious amounts of lemon juice and olive oil. Add salt and pepper to taste.

Nutrition Facts Per Serving: fat 9.1 g | Carbohydrate 47.2 g | Calories 398.1 | Protein 21 g

7. Sunrise Turmeric Tonic

Prep time: 5 mins, Cook time: 5 min, Servings: 2

Ingredients

- Turmeric powder 2 tsp
- Raw honey 2 tsp
- Ginger piece 1 inch grated
- Peppercorns 3-4
- Lemon sliced 1
- Hot water 2 cups (but not boiling)

Instructions

- Use a pestle to mash the turmeric, sugar, peppercorns, ginger, and lb to a pulp in a mortar.
- Then, evenly distribute the pasta among the serving mugs or glasses, garnish with lemon slices and a little water, and stir to combine.

Nutrition Facts Per Serving: fat 13.1 g | Carbohydrate 26 g | Calories 376.4 | Protein 27 g

8. Detox Wrap with Sunflower Seed Spread

Prep time: 5 mins, Cook time: 10 min, Servings: 6

Ingredients

Sunflower Seed Spread

- Socked sunflower seeds 1 cup
- Tomato 1
- Cilantro 1/4

- Sundried tomatoes 2-3
- Extra virgin oil 3 tbsp.
- Tahini 2 tbsp.
- Lemon juice 2
- Sea salt 1/4 tbsp.
- Black pepper 1/4 tbsp.

Wrap Toppings Options

- Sprouts as per your taste
- Cultured vegetables 1/4 cup
- Carrots shredded
- Red cabbage, sliced peppers etc.

Instructions

- Sunflower seeds that have been drained of water should be added to a food processor or blender. Blend in the remaining components until well combined. Add one or two tablespoons of water to achieve the desired consistency.
- To assemble the wrap, add 2 or 3 tbsp of spread. As desired, toppings can be added. Eat it by rolling it up.

Nutrition Facts Per Serving: fat 13.2 g | Carbohydrate 27.8 g | Calories 229 | Protein 21.9 g

9. Spaghetti Squash Hash Browns

Prep time: 15 mins, Cook time: 25 min, Servings: 6

Ingredients

- Spaghetti shredded squash 2 cups (about 1/2 small, cooked squash)
- Oil 1 tbsp.

Instructions

- Heat the oil in a nonstick skillet over medium heat.
- Utilizing paper towels, drain the squash of its water. 3. Use your hands to firmly press the

squash into tiny patties.

- Put the patties on the hot pan gently and cook them for 5 to 7 minutes on each side. If necessary, flip the food just once to achieve the desired browning.

- Serve while still warm after draining on paper towels.

Nutrition Facts Per Serving: fat 20 g | Carbohydrate 55 g | Calories 437 | Protein 16 g

10. Roasted Vegetable Salad for Hormone Balance

Prep time: 15 mins, Cook time: 25 min, Servings: 6

Ingredients

- Pumpkin seeds 1 tbsp. (lightly toasted)
- Pomegranate seeds 1
- Sweet potatoes 2
- Red bell pepper 1
- Carrots 2
- Yellow onion 1
- Cloves of garlic 4
- Kale leaves 3-4 (chopped)
- Fresh parsley 1 bunch (finely chopped)
- Quinoa 1/2 cup (uncooked)
- Apricots 2 dried (diced)
- Olive oil 1 tbsp.
- Cumin

Roasted Vegetable Salad Dressing

- Turmeric powder1 tsp
- Ginger 1 tsp (freshly grated)
- Lemon juice 2 tbsp. (freshly squeezed)

- Salt 1/2 tsp
- (Extra virgin) olive oil 2 tbsp.
- 1 pinch of ground black pepper
- Water 2 tbsp.
- Dijon mustard 2 tsp

Instructions

- Set the oven's temperature to 392°F/200°C. Put the baking sheet in the oven and preheat it to 350 degrees.
- Peel the potatoes, onions, and carrots and cut them into cubes to prepare the vegetables. Add chopped bell pepper to the baking sheet (baking). Add the cumin, drizzle some olive oil on top, and thoroughly toss to coat. The pan should be taken out of the oven after 20 minutes of baking.
- Prepare the quinoa while the vegetables are roasting. To rinse it, put it in a pot with water (1 cup). Over medium heat, boil; then, turn the heat down to low and simmer for 15 minutes. The pot should be turned off, covered, and left alone (the quinoa would absorb the steam and become fluffy).
- In a mixing bowl, combine the kale, parsley, and Quinoa with the roasted veggies, pumpkin, and pomegranate seeds.
- To create the dressing, combine all the ingredients in a jar, cover it, and shake briskly.
- Over the salad, drizzle the dressing, and toss to combine.

Nutrition Facts Per Serving: fat 7.9 g |Carbohydrate 58 g| Calories 467| Protein 14

11. Thai Cauliflower Rice Salad with Peanut Butter Sauce

Prep time: 20 mins, Cook time: 35 min, Servings: 6

Ingredients

For the salad

- Cauliflower 1 (head)
- Coconut milk 1 cup

- Onion 1 (diced)
- Garlic clove 2 (minced)
- Fresh parsley 1 (small bunch)
- Spring onions 2 (chopped)
- Almonds 1/4 cup (toasted chopped)
- Peeled mango 1 (small cubes)
- Bell pepper 1 (small cubes)
- Red cabbage ½ cup (chopped)
- Coconut oil 1 tsp

For the sauce

- Peanut butter 2 tbsp.
- Ginger peeled 1 inch
- Lime juice 2 tsp
- Raw honey 1 tsp
- Water 1/4 cup
- Sea salt 1/2 tsp

Instructions

- The cauliflower greens should be removed, divided into florets, rinsed, and well drained.
- In a food processor, blend or pulse the florets until they resemble rice in size.
- The garlic and onions are added to the hot coconut oil and cooked for one minute.
- Add the cauliflower and coconut milk, stir, and simmer for five minutes on low heat or until tender but not mushy.
- Please remove it from the fire and let it cool.
- Combine mango, cauliflower, bell pepper, spring onion, parsley, and red cabbage in a mixing dish.

- In a blender, combine the sauce ingredients and pulse until creamy and smooth.
- Pour over the cauli salad, then gently fold it in.
- Serve after adding fresh parsley and almonds as a garnish.

Nutrition Facts Per Serving: fat 23 g | Carbohydrate 29 g | Calories 347 | Protein 27 g

12. Tabbouleh

Prep time: 25 mins, Cook time: 20 min, Servings: 6

Ingredients

- Parsley bunch 1
- Mint bunch 1
- Lemon Juice 1
- Olive oil 2-3tbsp
- Bulgur wheat 50g
- Tomatoes 2 medium
- Red onion half

Instructions

- Bulgur wheat should be soaked in 100 ml of boiling water for five minutes or until the water has completely been absorbed.
- While doing so, finely cut the mint and parsley and slice the red onion and tomatoes.
- Combine the wheat with lemon juice, olive oil, herbs, onions, and tomatoes.

Nutrition Facts Per Serving: fat 8.1 g | Carbohydrate 49 g | Calories 411 | Protein 12.5 g

13. Vegetable stew

Prep time: 15 mins, Cook time: 15 min, Servings: 2

Ingredients

- Olive oil 1 tbsp.
- Peeled & sliced 1 onion
- Carrots 2 (peeled & diced)
- Parsnips 2(peeled & diced)
- Chopped celery stalks 2
- Swede 250g (peeled & diced)
- (1 pint hot) vegetable stock 600ml
- Can tomatoes 400g
- Can butter beans 420g
- Chopped parsley (handful)

Instructions

- The onion is cooked in a pan with hot oil over low heat for five minutes. The remaining veggies should be added, covered, and cooked over medium heat for 5 minutes or until they soften.
- Bring the stock and canned tomatoes to a boil, then lower the heat and cover the pan to maintain a simmer (for 10 mins). After adding the beans, cook the veggies for 5 minutes or until they are soft.
- Add chopped parsley as a garnish before serving.

Nutrition Facts Per Serving: fat 13 g | Carbohydrate 56 g | Calories 367 | Protein 24.7 g

14. Bliss Balls

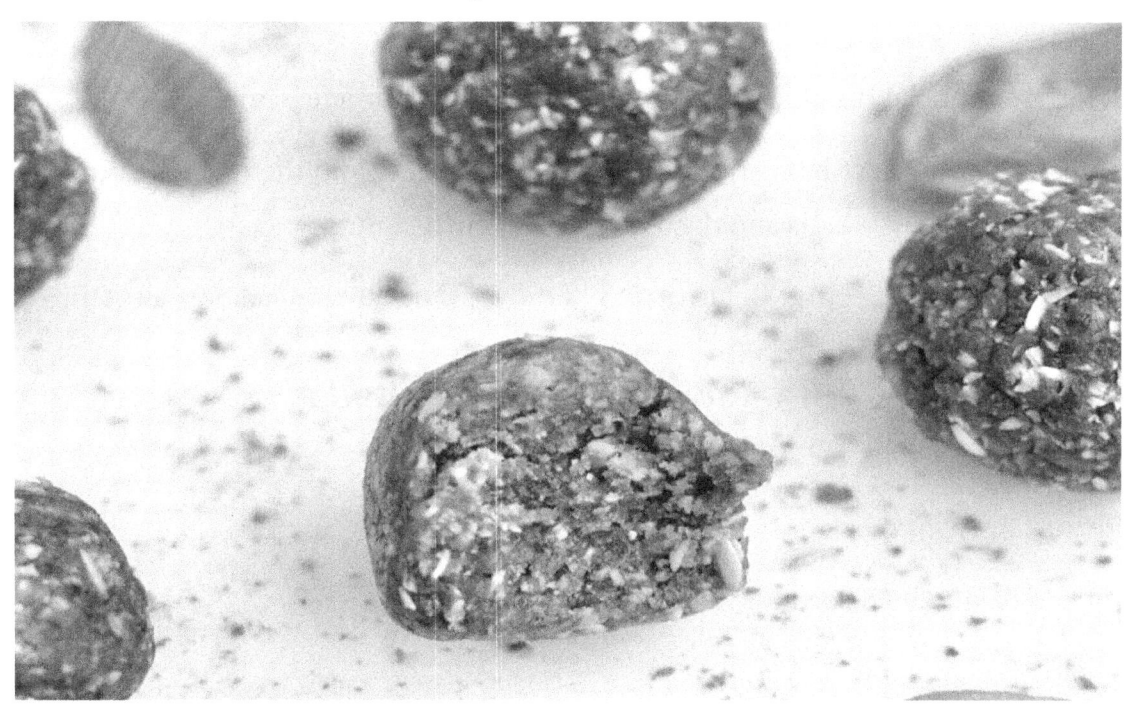

Prep time: 30 mins, Cook time: 05 mins, Servings: 3

Ingredients

- Four Medjool dates
- 1 cup of almond meal
- 1/2 cup of shredded coconut
- 1/3 cup of coconut oil
- 1/3 cup of cacao powder
- 1/3 cup of pistachios
- 1/4 cup of almonds
- 1 tbsp of chia seeds

Instructions

- Almonds and dates may be soaked in hot water to make them softer. Almonds should be soaked for at least four hours unless you have a powerful blender.
- Before letting the dates soften for about an hour, carefully remove the seed.

- Using a food processor, blender, or mixer, combine all the ingredients except the chocolate and chia seeds.
- Before serving, let the chia swell and soften in a bowl for a few minutes.
- Pistachios that aren't being utilized should be crushed, and the uncooked mixture should be formed into little balls and dusted with the crushed nuts.

Nutrition Facts Per Serving: Calories 328 | fat 8 g | Carbohydrates 28 g | Protein 34 g

15. Raw Cacao Energy Balls

Prep time: 20 mins, Cook time: 05 mins, Servings: 1

Ingredients

- 1/3 cup of shredded coconut
- 2 tbsp of coconut oil
- ½ cup of almonds
- 1/3 cup of cacao powder

Instructions

- The almonds should be blended to a fine powder. Grind them up fine.
- While blending, add the remaining ingredients. It should be simple to roll the dough into balls.
- Then, roll the dough onto balls using your preferred topping.
- You can eat them immediately or put them in the fridge overnight to harden them into balls.

Nutrition Facts Per Serving: Calories 405 | fat 8 g | Carbohydrates 43 g | Protein 26 g

16. Quinoa Bowl with Lentils and Mustard Vinaigrette

Prep time: 20 mins, Cook time: 30 min, Servings: 6

Ingredients

- Green lentils 1/2 cup
- Red quinoa 1/2 cup
- Kosher salt
- Red wine (vinegar) 2 tbsp.
- Lemon juice 1 tbsp.
- Dijon mustard 2 tsp
- Olive oil extra virgin 1/4 cup
- Black pepper (ground)
- Sliced celery stalks 3
- Green cabbage 2 cups (thinly sliced)
- Celery leaves 1 cup
- Mint leaves torn 1 cup

Instructions

- Lentils should be soft but maintain their form after 15 to 20 minutes of cooking lentils and quinoa in a big saucepan of salted boiling water. Place the drained food in a large mixing basin.
- Combine the mustard, vinegar, and lemon juice in a large mixing bowl. Slowly pour into the oil while swirling to create an emulsion. Add plenty of salt and pepper for seasoning. Toss the cabbage, celery stalks, mint, and celery leave with the lentils and quinoa to coat. Whenever necessary, add more salt and pepper to the dish.

Nutrition Facts Per Serving: fat 7.8 g | Carbohydrate 48 g | Calories 394 | Protein 17 g

17. Perfectly Roasted Sweet Potato Fries

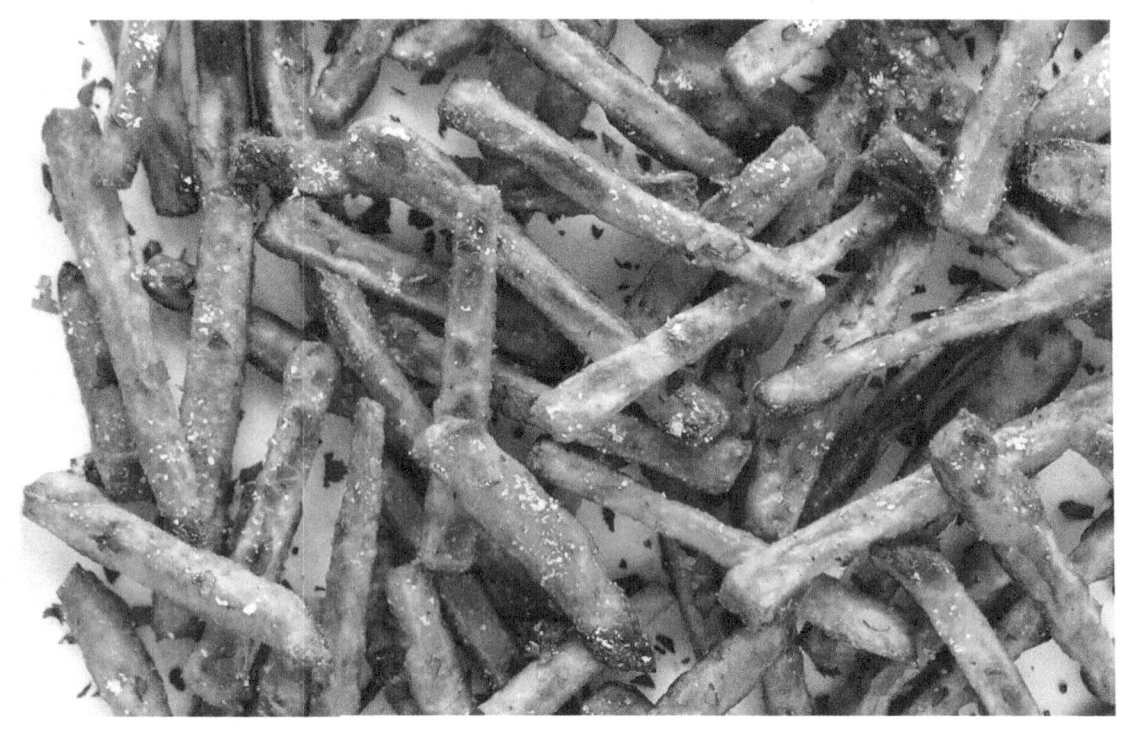

Prep time: 20 mins, Cook time: 40 min, Servings: 6

Ingredients

- Potatoes 3 (peeled & cut into fries' shape)
- Olive oil extra virgin 1 tbsp.
- Red chili flakes 1 tsp
- Salt 1/4 tsp
- For serving, add lime juice, diced red onion, chopped parsley, mashed avocado, and nutritional yeast

Instructions

- The oven should be preheated at 200 degrees Celsius, and parchment paper should be ready for a baking sheet.
- Sliced sweet potatoes should be placed in a big dish of cold water and soaked for fifteen minutes.
- With paper towels, thoroughly dry them after removing the water.
- Over that, put the cookie sheet.

- Sprinkle olive oil over the dish and spread it out evenly with your hands after seasoning it with salt and red chili flakes.
- Sweet potatoes should be arranged in a single layer, baked for fifteen minutes, turned over, and baked for ten minutes.
- Then, let it cool fully and keep it in a glass box for later use or take it out of the oven and serve it with the spices and dips.

Nutrition Facts Per Serving: fat 9.7 g | Carbohydrate 21.4 g | Calories 342 | Protein 16 g

18. Split Pea Soup with Coconut (Spiced)

Prep time: 25 mins, Cook time: 30 min, Servings: 8

Ingredients

Soup:

- Oil 2 tbsp.
- chopped red onion 1
- Chopped carrots 4
- Kosher salt
- Fennel seeds 1 tsp
- Curry powder Madras 2 tsp
- Mustard seeds 1 tsp
- Split peas (yellow) 12 oz
- Coconut & assembly:
- Coriander seeds 1/2 tsp
- Fennel seeds 1/2 tsp
- Mustard seeds 1/2 tsp
- Oil 2 tsp olive, vegetable, coconut, or olive
- Coconut flakes unsweetened 1/4 cup

- Kosher salt
- For serving, add Cilantro leaves

Instructions

The soup:

- Heat the oil in a large, heavy saucepan set over medium heat. Add the onion and carrots, sprinkle with a bit of salt, and simmer, often stirring, for approximately five minutes or until the veggies are very mushy and only have a slight color at the ends. Use a pestle and mortar to lightly crush or finely chop the fennel seeds. Curry, fennel seeds, and mustard seeds are cooked in a skillet with steady stirring for less than one minute until fragrant (mustard seeds will begin to explode). In a mixing bowl, add the separated peas, toss to coat, and then add enough water and stock to make four cups. For 50 to 55 minutes, or when the split peas are very mushy, and other peas are beginning to split, increase the heat to a low simmer, then bring to a boil, stirring regularly and adding additional water if the soup seems too thick.

- Use a potato masher to mash the soup until the split peas are tiny and the consistency is textured yet creamy (using an immersion for a smoother soup directly blend in the pot). If required, add more salt to the dish.

Assembly & amp; coconut:

- Lightly crush the fennel, mustard seeds, and cilantro while the soup is heating.

- Heat the oil in a low-temperature pan. Cook the spices and coconut flakes while stirring regularly for about a minute or until the coconut becomes golden brown and the spices start to crackle. Place on a dish, sprinkle with salt and let to cool (as it cools, the coconut will be crisp).

- On top of the soup, garnish with coriander and spiced coconut.

Nutrition Facts Per Serving: fat 8.8 g | Carbohydrate 18.9 g | Calories 364 | Protein 24.3 g

19. Miso-Harissa Delicate Squash And Brussels Sprouts Salad

Prep time: 15 mins, Cook time: 25 min, Servings: 6

Ingredients

- Trimmed Brussels sprouts 1/2 lb
- Delicata squash 1 lb
- Olive oil 1/4 cup
- White miso 1/4 cup
- Harissa pastes 1 tbsp.
- Honey 2 tsp
- Unseasoned rice vinegar 3 tbsp.
- Toasted chopped almonds 1/4 cup
- For serving, add Minced cilantro

Instructions

- Use parchment paper to line the baking sheet and preheat the oven to 205°C.
- It is best to chop Brussels sprouts in half lengthwise. Scrape out all the seeds after cutting your delicata squash in half lengthwise. Cut each half into half-moons that are one to two inches thick. You should apply the peel to the squash since it is edible.
- Mix the olive oil, harissa, miso, vinegar, and sugar in a mixing bowl. In a large mixing basin, combine the squash and Brussels sprouts with 1/3 cup of the harissa-miso combination. To uniformly coat the veggies, use your hands. Spread the veggies on the covered cookie sheet and roast them for 25 to 30 minutes, or until the Brussels sprouts are crisp and the squash is soft. About halfway through the cooking period, add the veggies.
- Heat a small dry pan over medium-high heat while the veggies cook. Cook the bread and almonds in the pan, occasionally stirring for 3 to 5 minutes, until golden brown. They should be taken out of the pan and put on the tray. Before finely cutting, let the mixture cool.
- Divide the steamed veggies, then top with chopped coriander and toasted almonds. Serve

with any remaining miso-harissa sauce.

- The miso-harissa sauce may be stored in the fridge for up to a week in an airtight container.

Nutrition Facts Per Serving: fat 15 g | Carbohydrate 34 g | Calories 356 | Protein 20 g

20. One-Pot Curried Cauliflower with Couscous and Chickpeas

Prep time: 15 mins, Cook time: 30 min, Servings: 6

Ingredients

- Virgin coconut oil (at room temperature) 3 tbsp.
- Chopped cauliflower head 1
- sliced red onion 1
- Chopped garlic cloves 3
- Curry powder 2 tsp
- Kosher salt 2 tsp
- Ground cumin 1 1/4 tsp
- The vegetable broth in low sodium 3 cups
- Chickpeas can be 1 (15.5-oz)
- Pearled couscous 1 cup
- Split red lentils 1/2 cup
- Limes 2 divided
- Coarsely cilantro leaves chopped 3 tbsp. Also, for serving, add whole leaves
- Baby spinach 5 oz
- For serving, add sliced almonds 1/4 cup

Instructions

- Heat two tablespoons of oil to medium heat in a big Dutch oven or saucepan. Cook the cauliflower in a pot for 5 to 8 minutes, turning periodically or until it is tender and gently browned. In a mixing dish, combine the garlic, onion, and 1 tbsp of the remaining oil. Add the oil and continue cooking the cauliflower and onion for five to seven minutes, stirring

- regularly. Cumin, salt, and curry powder should be added. Stirring often, cook for 30 seconds or until the spices are toasted.

- The broth should be heated through. For about 10 minutes, or until the couscous and lentils are thoroughly cooked, reduce the heat to low, add the couscous, chickpeas, and lentils, and occasionally stir to prevent the couscous from sticking. All the liquid has been transformed into a thick sauce.

- But three teaspoons are produced from one lime juice. In a mixing dish, combine the lime juice, cream, and three teaspoons. Slice the coriander thinly into a medium bowl. Add the water one spoonful until the sauce is thin enough to drizzle. If there are any extra limes, cut them into wedges.

- In a mixing dish, combine the spinach and chickpeas. Serve with lime wedges after covering with cilantro leaves and almonds.

Nutrition Facts Per Serving: fat 19 g | Carbohydrate 46 g | Calories 471 | Protein 25 g

21. Grain Bowl with Spiced Squash & Mushrooms

Prep time: 20 mins, Cook time: 45 min, Servings: 6

Ingredients

- White / brown rice barley 1/2 cup (red optional)

- Kosher salt

- Olive oil 3tbsp

- Black pepper 1/4 tsp

- Ground cinnamon 1/4 tsp

- Halved delicata squash, one medium

- Trimmed cremini/button mushrooms 8 oz

- Sliced 1/2" red onion 1

- Lemon juice 1 1/2 tsp

- Curry powder 1/4 tsp

- Baby greens (watercress/arugula) 2 cups

- For serving, add Lemon wedges & cilantro leaves

Instructions

- Set the oven's temperature to 205 Celsius. According to the directions on the packaging, prepare the grains with one or two tablespoons of salt.

- Then, using a fork, combine the oil, pepper, cinnamon, and 3/4 tsp salt in a large mixing bowl. Add the onion, squash, and mushrooms and toss to coat. Spread on a rimmed baking sheet, and roast for 25 to 30 minutes, turning halfway through, or until fork-tender veggies are gently browned.

- In a small mixing bowl, combine the curry powder, lemon juice, and 1/8 teaspoon salt. If required, divide the mixture into two bowls and swirl each bowl's surface—Layer the veggies and greens over the rice. Finish with coriander and, if preferred, a squeeze of lemon.

Nutrition Facts Per Serving: fat 8.6 g | Carbohydrate 27 g | Calories 318 | Protein 21.9 g

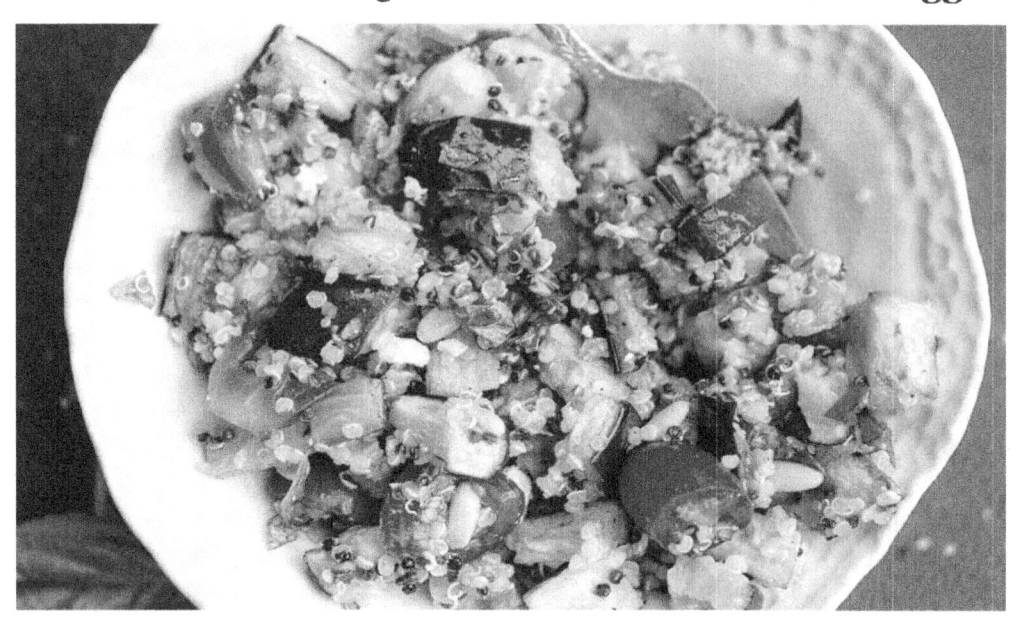

22. Mediterranean Quinoa Salad with Roasted Veggies

Prep time: 10 mins, Cook time: 20 min, Servings: 4

Ingredients

- Cooked quinoa 1 cup

- Diced yellow tomatoes 2

- Cherry tomatoes 5-7

- Small cubes of eggplant 1
- Red bell pepper in medium pieces 1
- Yellow onion 1 (cut into medium pieces)
- Dived cucumber 1
- Olive oil 2 tbsp.
- Sea salt 1/2 tsp
- Ground black pepper
- Basil leaves 5-6
- Oregano leaves 5-6
- Minced garlic cloves 2
- Apple cider vinegar 1 tsp
- Lemon juice 1 tbsp.
- Raw honey ½ tsp
- Toasted pine nuts 1 tbsp.

Instructions

- Set the oven to 175 Celsius for preheating.
- The aubergine, onion, and bell pepper should be placed on a cookie sheet lined with parchment paper. Add a little olive oil (about 1 tbsp) and season to taste.
- Afterward, remove the vegetables from the oven and set them aside to cool. For 20 minutes, roast.
- In a large mixing bowl, combine the cucumber, quinoa, garlic cloves, tomatoes, fresh spices, and roasted vegetables.
- To prepare the dressing, combine the remaining olive oil, honey, vinegar, and lemon juice in a mixing bowl.
- Pine nuts that have been toasted may be added before serving.

Nutrition Facts Per Serving: fat 9.4 g | Carbohydrate 23.7 g | Calories 281 | Protein 21.3 g

23. Cinnamon Carrot Sticks

Prep time: 10 mins, Cook time: 10 mins, Servings: 1

Ingredients

- One lb. peeled carrots
- A tbsp. of ground cinnamon
- 1 tbsp of Butter
- Pinch salt
- Double boiler

Instructions

- Vertically slice the carrots thinly.
- It just needs to steam for five minutes.
- Add the remaining ingredients to a boiler and bring it to a boil after draining the water.
- Lastly, cook the carrots in the butter over moderate heat until well coated (1-2 mins).

Nutrition Facts Per Serving: Calories 326 | fat 4 g | Carbohydrates 35 g | Protein 19 g

24. Foolproof Spinach & Feta Frittata

Prep Time: 10 mins, Cook Time: 15 mins, Serving: 2**Ingredients**

- 2 tsp of olive oil
- 1 peeled & finely sliced small brown onion
- 1 tsp garlic
- 251 g of baby spinach
- to taste Salt & pepper

Instructions

- Your grill's burners should be set to medium-high heat.
- Melt the butter in a medium-sized nonstick-coated frying pan and place it under the grill to crisp the outside.

- Cook the onion while occasionally stirring until it begins to soften and brown. Throw the spinach in and let it a moment to wilt. Allow the dish to cool completely after removing it from the heat source.

- Let the onion and spinach cool. To taste, add salt and pepper to the food.

- The frittata should be cooked and browned under the grill after 2 to 3 minutes.

- To release the frittata, place the plate on the pan and quickly but gently flip it over. Serve with a hot or cold, fresh salad on the side.

Nutrition Facts Per Serving: fat 15 g | Carbohydrate 35 g | Calories 436 | Protein 6 g

25. Lentil, Beetroot, & Hazelnut Salad along with Ginger Dressing

Prep Time: 10 mins, Cook Time: 10 mins, Serving: 2

Ingredients

- 1 cup rinsed Puy lentils
- 2 & ¾ cups water filtered
- salt Sea
- 3 beetroots cooked
- 2 finely sliced spring onions
- 2 tbsp chopped hazelnuts
- roughly chopped fresh mint, A handful
- roughly chopped fresh parsley A handful

Instructions

- In a saucepan, add the lentils and water. Bring to a boil, then lower the heat and simmer for 15-20 minutes, or until the liquid has been absorbed and the lentils are tender.

- Make a large bowl, put the lentils in it, and set it aside to cool.

- Add the beets, spring onions, hazelnuts, and herbs after the lentil dish has simmered for a while.

- Whisk together the ginger, oil, mustard, & vinegar in your bowl to create the dressing.

- Before serving, drizzle the salad with the dressing.

Nutrition Facts Per Serving: Calories 391 | fat 17 g | Carbohydrate 52 g | Protein 12 g

26. Tofu Curry

Prep Time: 25 Mins, Cook Time: 2 Hrs, Serving: 4

Ingredients:

- 2 cup green bell pepper, diced
- 1 cup firm tofu, cut into cubes
- 1 onion, peeled and diced
- What you'll need from the store cupboard:
- 1 ½ cups canned coconut milk
- 1 cup tomato paste
- 2 cloves garlic, diced fine
- 2 tbsp. raw peanut butter
- 1 tbsp. garam masala
- 1 tbsp. curry powder
- 1 ½ tsp salt

Instructions:

- Add all the ingredients except the tofu to a blender or food processor. Process until everything is well-combined.
- Add the tofu after pouring it into a slow cooker—cover and cook for two hours on high.
- Serve over cauliflower rice after thoroughly mixing.

Nutrition Facts Per Serving: Calories 389 | fat 28 g | Carbohydrates 20 g | Protein 13 g

27. Easy and Yummiest Kulfi Recipe

Prep Time: 10 mins, cook time: 8 hrs, Serving: 12

Ingredients

- 2 cans of milk evaporated
- 2 cans table cream canned
- 1 can condensed milk sweetened
- 2 white bread slices
- ¼ tsp cardamom ground
- 12 almonds blanched

Instructions

- Condensed milk and cream evaporated milk are combined in a blender to create breadcrumbs for a pudding. Cardamom and almonds should be combined and processed in a food processor or blender for 3–4 minutes or until smooth. Freeze for eight hours or overnight in a glass dish. Slice the dish into squares to serve.

Nutrition Facts Per Serving: fat 16 g | Carbohydrate 23 g | Calories 256 | Protein 5 g

28. Guacamole

Prep Time: 20 Mins, Cook Time: 0 Mins, Servings: 1

Ingredients

- Ripe avocados
- Diced onion
- 2 tomatoes, diced
- Lime juice
- Pinch salt

Instructions

- Once the avocados have been peeled, and the pits removed, slice them.
- In a mixing bowl, add the pieces and mash them until entirely smooth.

- Add the remaining ingredients and whisk well.

Nutrition Facts Per Serving: Calories 345 | fat 7 g | Carbohydrates 42 g | Protein 23 g

29. Homemade Lunch Combination

Prep Time: 10 mins, Cook Time: 10 mins, Serving: 1

Ingredients

- 6 crackers wheat
- 1 romaine torn lettuce leaf
- 1 sliced Roma tomato

Instructions

- Put hummus and crackers in an airtight container. Storage options for the Cheddar vegetable include zip-top plastic bags. Create a second zip-top plastic bag to hold the lettuce and tomato.
- Add lettuce and tomato to the wheat crackers after that.

Nutrition Facts Per Serving: fat 9.7 g | Carbohydrate 18 g | Calories 296 | Protein 25 g

Chapter 4: Dinner Recipes

After a hectic workday a dinner full of nutrients will restore your drained energy. This chapter includes nutrient rich dinner recipes.

1. Portobello mushroom burgers

Prep time: 20 mins, Cook time: 15 min, Servings: 4

Ingredients

- Portobello mushroom caps 6 large
- Avocado oil 4 tbsp.
- Agave syrup 2 tbsp.
- Essential lime juice 2 tbsp.
- Extra veggies: onions, bell peppers, mushrooms, etc.
- Sea salt & Cayenne pepper

Instructions

- Start by combining the marinade ingredients in a dish to make the portobello mushroom burgers.
- Put the mushroom caps in a baking dish, and then cover them with your marinade. For approximately 30 minutes, let the mushrooms marinate in the marinade, scraping the tops, as necessary.
- Start grilling your mushrooms with the cap side down for 5 to 7 minutes on each side. As the mushrooms cook, start coating them with the marinade.
- Serve topped with various ingredients or mixed veggies.

Nutrition Facts Per Serving: fat 12.8 g | Carbohydrate 39 g | Calories 294 | Protein 24 g

2. Magic green falafels

Prep time: 15 mins, Cook time: 30 min, Servings: 6

Ingredients

- Garbanzo beans dry 2 cups
- Chopped onion 1 large
- Chopped red bell pepper 1/3 cup
- Fresh basil 2/3 cup
- Fresh dill 1/2 cup
- Sea salt 1 tsp.
- Oregano 1/4 tsp.
- Garbanzo bean flour 1/2 cup
- For frying Grapeseed/ avocado oil

Instructions

- Cooking the chickpeas until they are soft is the first step in making the Magic Green Falafels. After draining the beans, rinse them.
- Add the other ingredients to the food processor along with the chickpeas. An onion, fresh herbs, red bell pepper, sea salt, flour, and oregano are among the components.
- All ingredients should be finely chopped, and a coarse meal should develop after many pulses. Once the texture resembles a good meal, scrape off the edges and re-pump. If necessary, adjust the seasonings.
- The ingredients should be added to a big bowl. Create thick cubes or tiny balls with your fingers, then arrange them on the board covered in parchment paper. Before serving, place in the fridge for at least one hour.
- Over medium heat, add oil to a wide skillet until it is about an inch deep, and cook for 5-7 minutes. The miraculous Green Falafels are fried on each side for 2 to 3 minutes once the oil is hot.

Nutrition Facts Per Serving: fat 14.3 g | Carbohydrate 44 g | Calories 334 | Protein 22 g

3. Roast tomato and orange soup recipe

Prep time: 15 mins, Cook time: 35 min, Servings: 2

Ingredients

- Tomatoes 900g
- Chopped 2 garlic cloves
- Olive oil 4 tbsp.
- Diced onions 2
- Carrots peeled/scrubbed 2
- Diced celery sticks 1
- Hot vegetable stock 560ml
- Orange juice 100ml
- For serving the zest of 1 small orange
- (optional) Edible flowers

Instructions

- Set the oven's temperature to 160°C or 180°C (gas/fan mark 4).
- Arrange the tomatoes on a large baking pan and scatter the chopped garlic. Add two tablespoons of olive oil, salt, and black pepper to season. The oven is hot; after placing the tomatoes in the oven, roast them for 45 minutes, stirring once.
- After stirring the tomatoes, warm the remaining olive oil in a large, deep pan over low heat for 20 minutes while sautéing the carrots, onions, and celery. Add the roasted tomatoes and garlic. Return to the pan and stir briefly before adding the orange juice and stock to the tank.
- After simmering for one to two minutes, remove the soup and let it cool before liquidizing. Adding the skillet. After returning the soup to the pot, taste it for seasoning and, if required, season it with additional salt and black pepper. Ensure it's hot enough if you intend to serve it straight away.
- Let the soup cool fully before transferring it to a big container and chilling it for a few hours

if you're serving it cold.

- Serve with orange zest and edible flowers like nasturtium or borage.

Nutrition Facts Per Serving: fat 13 g | Carbohydrate 37 g | Calories 361 | Protein 24 g

---

4. Green Detox Smoothie Bowl

Prep time: 20 mins, Cook time: 30 min, Servings: 2

Ingredients

- Fresh spinach leaves 1/2 cup
- Fresh parsley 1 small bunch
- Lemon juice 1/2 tbsp.
- Almond butter 1 tbsp.
- Pineapple 1/2 cup
- Chia seeds 2 tsp
- Purified water 1 1/2 cup
- Low-fat coconut milk 1/2 cup
- Desiccated coconut flakes 1 unsweetened mixed, nuts & seeds

Instructions

- All ingredients should be combined in a mixer and processed until smooth to create a creamy beverage.
- Before serving, spread in serving bowls and top with seeds, coconut flakes, and pollen.

Nutrition Facts Per Serving: fat 9.7 g | Carbohydrate 29 g | Calories 294 | Protein 21 g

5. Alkaline Lasagne

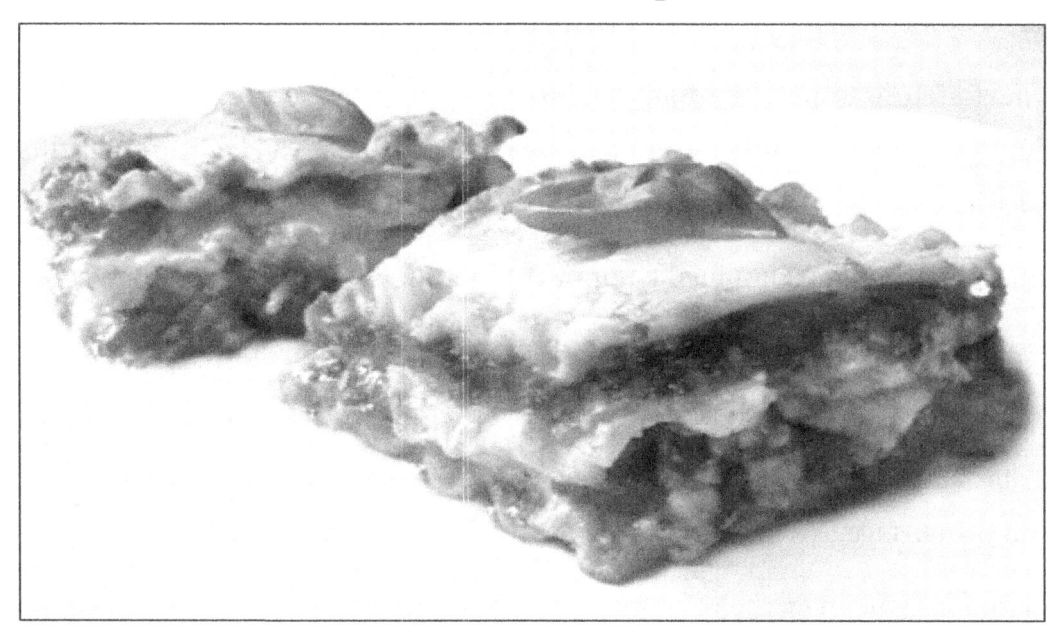

Prep time: 10 mins, Cook time: 50 min, Servings: 2

Ingredients

- Spelled Lasagne
- 2 handfuls of baby spinach
- 1 pack of soft tofu
- 1 aubergine
- 1 courgette
- 2 cloves of garlic
- 8 Roma tomatoes
- Handful fresh basil
- 1 red pepper
- 1 red onion
- 1 lemon

Instructions

- Set the oven to 180 degrees. The red pepper's skin may be removed by roasting it until it

- starts to burn, placing it on a plate, then cling-film-covering until it is cool enough to handle. After a few minutes, throw away the cling film and then peel the peel away.

- The next step is to peel the four tomatoes, which may be done by submerging them in boiling water for one to two minutes. Use a sharp knife to slice through the skin of the tomatoes as you remove them. It should be simple to remove the skin.

- Sauce made from the combined components should be kept in a separate container.

- To prepare a second sauce, combine the spinach, tofu, and lemon juice.

- The courgette and aubergine should be taken off the grill, sprinkled with a bit of salt, and let rest for five minutes before being cut. After the required time, gently pat any moisture still on the surface. No matter what, skipping this step would result in too mushy lasagne.

- Layer the lasagne over the tofu and spinach, then the courgette and aubergine. Pour the pepper and tomato sauce on top after you've reached the top of the dish. After cooking for 35 to 40 minutes, serve with a green salad.

Nutrition Facts Per Serving: Calories 360|fat 17 g | Carbohydrate 45 g| Protein 15 g

6. Kale Detox Salad with Pesto

Prep time: 20 mins, Cook time: 30 min, Servings: 5

Ingredients

Carrot Top Pesto

- Bunch Carrots 1 Top
- Extra Virgin Olive Oil 1/4 Cup
- Salt 1/4 Tsp
- Pepper 1/4 Tsp
- 1/2 Lemon Juice from

Roasted Veg

- Fingerling 1 lb. Potatoes cut in rounds
- Purple Carrots 3-4 Large cut-in rounds
- Chickpeas 1 15 oz. Can drain & rinse

- Olive Oil Drizzle
- Salt 1 Tsp
- Pepper 1 Tsp
- Dried Parsley 1 Tsp
- Dried Basil 1 Tsp
- Garlic Powder 1/2 Tsp
- Dried Thyme Few Sprinkles

Rest Salad

- Lacinato Kale Sliced Thin
- Cooked Brown Rice 1 Cup
- If desired, Sliced Jalapeño
- Sesame Seeds, if desired

Instructions

- Set the oven's temperature to 425 degrees Fahrenheit.
- Clean and dry the carrots and potatoes to prepare the vegetables. Discs that are ¼ inch broad should be separated from each other.
- Cut-up carrots, chickpeas, and potatoes should all be combined in a mixing bowl. Mix the spices and olive oil in a mixing bowl and stir to coat everything evenly.
- The vegetables and chickpeas should be baked for 45 to 50 minutes on a baking sheet coated with parchment paper. Please remove it from the oven and put it aside to cool after they are finished cooking.
- To prepare the pesto, combine all the ingredients in a food processor and process them quickly until the pesto is smooth before prepping the vegetables.
- In a bowl, combine the pesto and the Lacinato kale, ensuring the kale is well covered. Next, incorporate the roasted veggies with brown rice and chickpeas. Check to see that it is well mixed before combining it.
- Sesame seeds may be placed on top of the meals before serving.

Nutrition Facts Per Serving: fat 18.4 g | Carbohydrate 34 g | Calories 317 | Protein 9.8 g

7. Detox rainbow roll-ups with peanut sauce

Prep time: 20 mins, Cook time: 25 min, Servings: 4

Ingredients

Rainbow roll-ups:

- Carrots,
- Cucumbers,
- Curry hummus
- Red cabbage
- Cooked rice/quinoa (optional)
- Cilantro and peanuts
- Collard greens

Peanut sauce:

- Peanut butter 3/4 cup
- Soy sauce 1/4 cup (tamari/coconut aminos
- Rice vinegar 1/4 cup
- Water 1/4 cup
- Honey 2 tbsp
- Clove garlic 1

Instructions

- To prepare, slice off just enough of the collard leaf's stem or spine to make it flexible rather than removing it.
- Roll up: Spread the fillings out on a collard leaf and do so. Maintaining order, fold the ends and move them from front to back.
- To prepare the peanut sauce, combine all the ingredients in a food processor or blender.

Nutrition Facts Per Serving: fat 11.3 g | Carbohydrate 28 g | Calories 341 | Protein 21 g

8. Comforting Cashew Curry

Prep time: 25 mins, Cook time: 30 min, Servings: 6

Ingredients

- Coconut milk 1/2 13.5-oz can
- Water 1/4 cup
- Green beans 1 cup trimmed
- Large carrots 2 chopped
- Chopped cauliflower 1 cup
- Red bell pepper 1 chopped
- Onion 1 large chopped
- Minced garlic cloves 3
- Minced ginger 1 tbsp./ground ginger 1 tsp
- Curry pastes 1 tsp
- Cayenne optional 1/2 tsp
- For garnish cashews, 1/2 cup
- For garnish cilantro 1/2 bunch

Instructions

- Except for the cilantro and cashews, combine all the ingredients in a big saucepan. Cook the vegetables for 10 to 15 minutes until they are fragrant and soft. Serve it after taking it off the heat. Garnish cilantro and cashews in each bowl.

Nutrition Facts Per Serving: fat 19.2 g | Carbohydrate 46 g | Calories 295 | Protein 16.7 g

9. Spicy Carrot & Greens

Prep time: 15 mins, Cook time: 0 min, Servings: 2

Ingredients

- 1 broccoli, large
- 2 carrots
- 6 brussels sprouts
- 2 garlic cloves
- 1 tsp caraway seeds
- 1 lemon
- 1/2 lemon
- Olive oil

Instructions

- Cut the broccoli into bite-sized pieces and slice the brussels sprouts. Cook the vegetables in light steam for 5-8 minutes.
- Once the steaming is complete, chop the garlic and reheat it in a skillet with the caraway seeds, lemon peel, and lemon juice.
- After a brief period of heating, add the carrots and brussels sprouts.

Nutrition Facts Per Serving: Calories 416|fat 19 g | Carbohydrate 48 g| Protein 13.3 g

10. Roasted Cauliflower Detox Bowl with Tahini Sauce

Prep time: 20 mins, Cook time: 35 min, Servings: 6

Ingredients

Bowls

- Large Kale leaves 3
- Clove garlic 1
- Quinoa 1/2 cup (dry weight)

- Red cabbage 1/4
- Avocado 1
- Large cauliflower 1/2
- Olive oil 1 tsp
- Ground cumin 1/4 tsp
- Cress

Tahini sauce

- Head garlic roasted 1
- raw cashews 1/2 cup soaked overnight in water
- Tahini 2 tbsp.
- Water 4-6 tbsp.
- Kosher salt 1/4-1/2 tsp

Instructions

- Turn the oven's temperature up to 200 degrees. Cauliflower florets should be mixed with olive oil and powdered cumin: for 20 to 25 minutes or until browned and roasted.
- To prepare the sauce, combine all the ingredients in a food processor except the salt and water. Add a little water while blending until the sauce is smooth. Add additional water and process the sauce until it is as smooth as the food processor will allow. Scrape down the edges, as necessary. To taste, add salt to the dish.
- Quinoa should be boiled for 10 minutes, drained, and left aside. Meanwhile, thinly slice the kale and red cabbage, and sauté in a skillet with minced garlic until wilted. To make sure the quinoa is evenly distributed, toss it in.
- Put part of the kale combination in the bottom of the bowl, then add the roasted cauliflower, sliced avocado, drizzled tahini sauce, and optionally some cress on top.

Nutrition Facts Per Serving: fat 9.9 g | Carbohydrate 27.4 g | Calories 329 | Protein 12.8 g

11. Easy Veggie Wrap with Avocado and Halloumi

Prep time: 20 mins, Cook time: 15 min, Servings: 2

Ingredients

- Large tortilla 2 wraps gluten-free/whole-wheat
- Avocado peeled 1, stone removed
- Halloumi sliced 4 oz. in ½" pieces
- Fresh spinach 1 cup
- Bell peppers 2
- Small red onion 1 diced
- Walnut kernel halves 4 (about 10 g) crushed
- Vinegar 1 tbsp.
- Extra virgin olive oil 2 tsp
- Lemon juice 1 tbsp.
- Dijon mustard 1 tbsp.
- Salt 1/2 tsp

Instructions

- Fire up the grill.
- With a fork, mash the avocado in a medium bowl. Add 1 teaspoon of lemon juice, stir, and leave aside.
- To prepare the creamy dressing, put the mustard, olive oil, salt, and lemon juice in a small pot, cover it, and shake briskly.
- Grill slices of halloumi cheese and bell peppers. Halloumi should be fried for three minutes, flipped over, and cooked for another three minutes. Rotate the red peppers until they are evenly cooked on each side (about 15 mins).
- Halloumi should be taken from the grill and put in a bowl.
- Bell peppers should be peeled from the grill, their stems and seeds removed, and then sliced

into strips. Placed aside in a basin and covered with vinegar.

- Keep the grill on a low heat setting until the wraps are done.
- To make the wraps, spread half an avocado mash on a tortilla, leaving a 1-inch circle off the hand.
- Add a couple of dressings, then some spinach leaves.
- Add the well-drained vinegar, half of the pepper slices, and more spinach leaves.
- Place half of the red onion, crumbled walnuts, and halloumi slices on top.
- Add a few additional dressing drops, then wrap the items.
- They should be grilled for two minutes on each side.
- Slice in half after removing from the grill and serve right away.
- Skip the seasoning and cover them in plastic if you won't be eating them straight away. Until you're ready to grill it, keep it in the fridge. It might last for as long as two days.

Nutrition Facts Per Serving: fat 18.2 g | Carbohydrate 39.1 g | Calories 423 | Protein 29 g

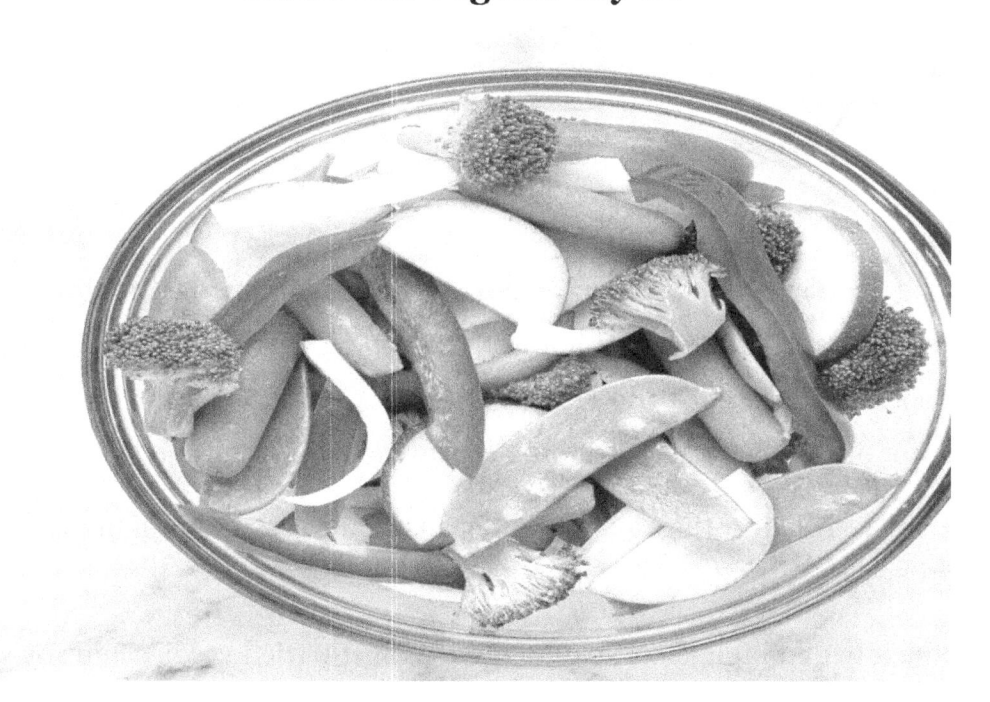

12. Seven-veg stir-fry 20

Prep time: 30 mins, Cook time: 15 min, Servings: 1

Ingredients

- Thai rice noodles 250g pack
- Groundnut oil 1-2 tbsp.
- Red pepper 1, deseeded & cut into thumb-length strips
- 2.5cm fresh root ginger (1in) piece, peeled & cut into slivers
- Baby sweetcorn 8, halved lengthways
- Carrots 2 medium, peeled & cut in batons
- Asparagus tip 8
- Mini sugar-snap peas/mange tout 3½ oz.
- Sweet chili dipping sauce 4tbsp/hoisin sauce
- Optional red chili 1, deseeded & chopped finely
- Pak choi 2 heads, quartered lengthways
- Fresh beansprouts 100g/150g pack
- Spring onions 4-6, trimmed & thinly sliced
- Mint & coriander leaves, chopped roughly
- To serve Soy sauce

Instructions

- Place the noodles in a large bowl and cover them with enough boiling water. Give it five minutes. In a large frying pan or hot wok, add 1 tablespoon of oil and stir-fry the ginger and red pepper for 30 seconds while the veggies cook. Add the mange tout or sugar snaps and stir-fry for one minute before adding the asparagus, carrots, and sweetcorn.
- Pack Choi, red chili, spring onions, and beansprouts are added, along with 4 tbsp of water, and the mixture is cooked for a short while.
- Combine it with mint and coriander. Serve with stir-fried veggies and soy sauce on top for flavor.

Nutrition Facts Per Serving: fat 14.6 g | Carbohydrate 37.2 g | Calories 382 | Protein 21.3 g

13. Alkaline Cous-Cous

Prep time: 15 mins, Cook time: 0 min, Servings: 2

Ingredients

- 2 servings of couscous (according to packet)
- 1 handful of spinach
- 1 avocado
- 2 tomatoes
- Half chopped pepper
- Seasonal herbs
- 1 lemon or lime, juiced
- avocado oil /olive/Udo's Choice

Instructions

- The veggies should be chopped up and placed on top of the couscous. Juice and oil should be adjusted to taste.
- This recipe might be more filling by using gently cooked green vegetables such as fine beans, broccoli, sugar snap peas, or any other form of greens.

Nutrition Facts Per Serving: Calories 406|fat 18 g | Carbohydrate 46 g| Protein 18 g

14. Thai Green Curry Made Alkaline

Prep time: 20 mins, Cook time: 30 min, Servings: 2

Ingredients

- 2 spring onions
- Broccoli
- 1/4 cauliflower
- 1 carrot sliced
- 125ml of coconut milk

- Handful coriander
- Large finger of ginger
- 1 stick of lemongrass
- 1-2 chilies
- 2 limes
- 1 tsp green curry paste
- Cubes of firm tofu (optional)
- Soba noodles or brown rice.

Instructions

- Before adding them to the lime juice, cut the coriander finely, slice the ginger, and crush the chopped lemongrass chili. Serve right away. After combining the ingredients, infuse.
- You may also slice the broccoli or cauliflower into smaller pieces and sauté them together with Asian greens or tofu, if you want, in addition to slicing the veggies.
- After five minutes, add the coconut milk, paste, lime, lemongrass, integrated chili, and lime to the cooked veggies.
- After boiling for five minutes, serve over brown rice or soba noodles.

Nutrition Facts Per Serving: Calories 360|fat 13 g | Carbohydrate 31 g| Protein 19 g

15. Alkaline Lunchtime Wraps

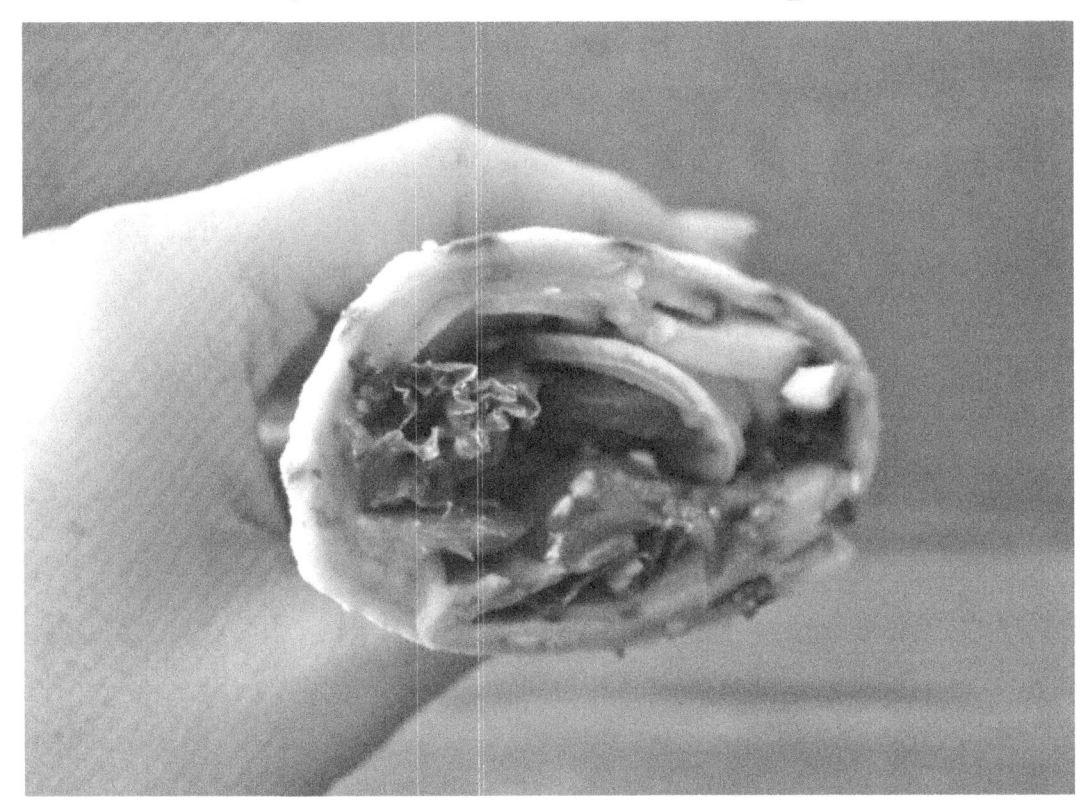

Prep time: 10 mins, Cook time: 0 min, Servings: 2

Ingredients

- 1/3 cucumber
- Lettuce leaves
- 1 tomato
- Handful spinach leaves
- Sunflower seeds
- Hummous
- tortillas/wraps (Wheat-free)
- ¼ lemon

Instructions

- Salad components should be well-washed and cubed to make wrapping them simpler.
- Spread the hummus on the wrap just to the left of the center.

- Put the wrap together first, spread the hummus with the seeds and add the salad ingredients.
- Fold the bottom length first, then securely wrap and tuck it up to prevent spills.

Nutrition Facts Per Serving: Calories 286|fat 11 g | Carbohydrate 32 g| Protein 14 g

16. Kale Slaw & Creamy Dressing

Prep time: 15 mins, Cook time: 0 min, Servings: 2

Ingredients

- 1 bunch of kale (any variety)
- 4 cups red cabbage, shredded
- 1 red onion
- 1 bell pepper (capsicum)
- 1/3 cup of sunflower seeds
- 1/2 bunch of coriander
- 1/4 cup of sesame seeds
- 1-inch piece of root ginger

For dressing:

- 1 cup raw cashews (soaked overnight)
- 1 cup vegetable stock
- 1 garlic clove

Instructions

- Before adding the dressing, combine the kale, red cabbage, bell pepper, onion, coriander seeds, and ginger in a large salad bowl.
- The following ingredients should be put in a high-speed blender and processed until smooth to make the cashew dressing. A warmer dressing may be made using heated stock, or the stock can chill and then be added. If you have a powerful blender, there is no need to let the cashews soak all night.

- The slaw will be combined once the dressing has been added. If necessary, add additional stock or cashews to alter the consistency.

Nutrition Facts Per Serving: Calories 336|fat 18 g | Carbohydrate 53 g| Protein 21 g

17. GABA rice + a Mental-Health Supporting Bowl

Prep time: 20 mins, Cook time: 25 min, Servings: 8

Ingredients

For the GABA rice

- Organic brown rice 2/3 cup
- Purified water 3 cups

For the Nourishing Bowl

- Red cabbage sauerkraut 1/2 cup
- Bunches fresh parsley 2 large
- Yellow onion 1/2, diced
- Portobello mushrooms 8 cuts in slices
- Avocado oil 1 tsp
- Salt 1/4 tsp
- Black pepper Freshly ground
- Extra virgin olive oil 1 tbsp.
- Fresh lime juice 1 tbsp.

Instructions

- Rinse the brown rice well and place it in a bowl. Drain it first, then cover it with water.
- Set the bowl aside to soak for 24 hours at room temperature and cover it with a lid or large plate. Drain and thoroughly clean the water if it stinks before adding more water.
- At room temperature, let the rice germinate. To keep the grains moist, periodically mist the rice with filtered water. After 48 hours, there could be a few tiny sprouts on the rice grains.
- Cook the rice until fluffy and soft for 20 minutes on low heat with 1 1/2 cups of filtered

water.

- Fry the mushrooms in the same skillet as you sauté the mushrooms in avocado oil over medium heat.

- Finely chop the parsley and mix it with the onion in a medium bowl to form the parsley salad. In a mixing dish, combine the olive oil, salt, pepper, and lemon juice.

- Serve the heated mushroom, rice, and parsley salad on the sauerkraut in serving bowls.

Nutrition Facts Per Serving: fat 10.8 g | Carbohydrate 37 g | Calories 372 | Protein 11 g

18. Aubergine & black bean Alkaline Chili

Prep time: 35 mins, Cook time: 20 min, Servings: 2

Ingredients

- Olive or coconut oil
- 200g of aubergine, cubes
- 1 red onion, chopped
- 2 cloves of garlic, crushed
- 5 red chilies, chopped
- Ground cinnamon
- 400g tin of tomatoes (organic)
- 1/2 tsp of ground coriander
- ground cumin
- 250g of black beans, cooked
- Sea salt
- Black pepper, freshly ground

Instructions

- The cumin seeds and onions should be browned for two minutes in medium-high heat coconut oil.

- The remaining potato slices, chickpeas, aubergine, ground coriander, turmeric, and cumin should then be added. After three more minutes of cooking, turn off the heat.

- You can now make the sauce. Before adding the chopped tomatoes, turmeric, other spices, and savories, immediately add the garlic, onion, ginger, and cloves to the skillet and sauté for 60 seconds. Increase the amount of coconut oil in the pan. Allow things to develop during the next three minutes.

- In a hand mixer, mash the sauces together roughly (or large blender). Add the vegetables, coriander, water, and any more salt or pepper to taste before mixing everything.

- You need to cook for 20 minutes to be ready. Garnish with fresh coriander and serve with brown rice!

Nutrition Facts Per Serving: Calories 387|fat 10 g | Carbohydrate 37 g| Protein 18 g

19. Stir-fry mushroom and broccoli

Prep time: 10 mins, Cook time: 25 min, Servings: 8

Ingredients

- Cayenne pepper corn flour pinch 1 tbsp.
- Soy sauce spray oil 2 tbsp. for frying
- Unsalted cashew nuts 25g
- Shiitake mushrooms 120g halved
- Broccoli 200g, chopped in florets
- Clove garlic 1, crushed
- Ginger root 1 small piece, finely chopped
- Spring onions 2, diagonally sliced
- Rice wine 4 tbsp.

Instructions

- Mix the corn flour and cayenne in a mixing bowl and secure the lid. Add the soy sauce and stir. Let sit in an excellent area for 30 minutes.

- Cashews should be stir-fried for 30 seconds or until golden brown and then transferred to a serving platter. Spray a wok with oil and heat it over high heat.

- Mushrooms should then be added and cooked for 1-2 minutes or until golden. They should be cooked for 1-2 minutes or until they turn pink. Add the remaining ingredients and stir for an additional minute.

- Re-add the nuts to the pan, increase the heat to medium, add the rice wine and some water, cover the pan, and simmer for an additional minute. Serve with glass noodles or cooked rice.

Nutrition Facts Per Serving: fat 14.9 g | Carbohydrate 38 g | Calories 389.9 | Protein 23.5 g

20. Grilled mackerel with chili, orange, lemon, and watercress

Prep time: 10 mins, Cook time: 15 min, Servings: 5

Ingredients

- Crushed black peppercorns 1 tsp
- Ground coriander 2 tsp
- Lemon zest finely grated 1 tbsp.
- Oranges 4
- Red chili 1, deseeded & finely chopped
- Mackerel fillets 8 x 150g (not smoked)
- Chopped coriander 2 tbsp.
- Watercress 110g
- Red onion 1 small, peeled & thinly sliced

Instructions

- Warm up the grill. In a mixing bowl, combine the black peppercorns, lemon zest, and coriander powder. Grate half an orange and add it to the coriander mixture and half of the minced red chili.

- Apply the mixture after gently rupturing the mackerel skin. Cook the mackerel for five minutes, or until it is crisp and cooked, with the skin-side up on the grill rack. Before serving, add the cilantro that has been chopped.

- Oranges should be cut into pieces. Each orange's top and bottom should be removed, followed by the peel and any remaining white pith, all using a thin, sensitive knife. To free it, cut down each side of each segment.

- In four servings, orange segments, red onion that have been diced, and the leftover chili are placed on top of the watercress. Top with grilled mackerel when serving.

Nutrition Facts Per Serving: fat 13.4 g | Carbohydrate 41.6 g | Calories 387 | Protein 19 g

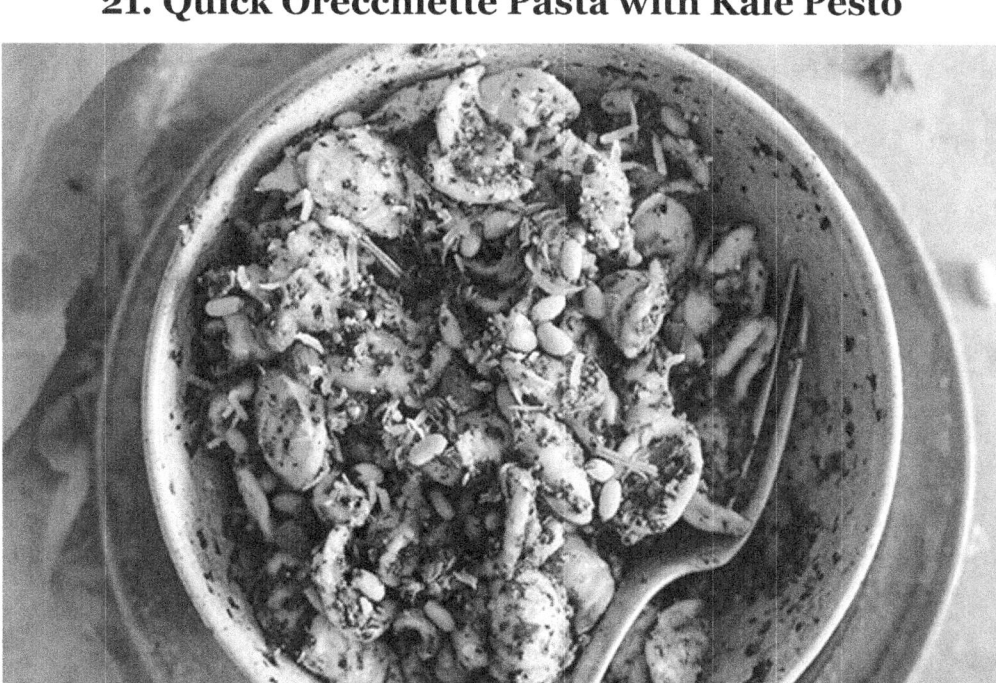

21. Quick Orecchiette Pasta with Kale Pesto

Prep time: 15 mins, Cook time: 25 min, Servings: 2

Ingredients

- Fresh Kale 1 bunch chopped
- Bunch fresh basil 1 small
- Sage leaves 2 fresh
- Garlic clove 3
- Toasted pine nuts 1 cup
- Extra virgin olive oil 2 tbsp.
- Dijon mustard 1 tsp
- Red chili flakes 1/2 tsp

- Lemon 1/2 juice
- Sea salt Pinch
- Orecchiette pasta 1/2 box 2 cups
- Fresh lemon juice, toasted pine nuts, and red chili flakes to garnish:

Instructions

- Mix the fresh herbs, garlic, lemon juice, and olive oil in a mixing bowl. Pulse the ingredients several times to create a mash.
- Pulse a few times to blend after adding the salt, pine nuts, Dijon, and chili flakes.
- Put the mixture in a container with a lid.
- Follow the directions for cooking the orecchiette.
- Three tablespoons of fresh pesto should be added to the big mixing bowl and well mixed.
- Into bowls, divide the mixture. Before serving, add fresh lemon juice and extra virgin olive oil, season with red chili flakes and toast the pine nuts.

Nutrition Facts Per Serving: fat 21 g | Carbohydrate 49 g | Calories 399 | Protein 26 g

22. Vegetarian Pizza with Autumn Toppings

Prep time: 15 mins, Cook time: 10 min, Servings: 2

Ingredients

For the Crust

- Whole wheat flour 2/3 cups
- Dried yeast 1/2 tbsp.
- Brown sugar 2 tsp
- Extra virgin olive oil 1 tbsp.
- Warm water 2/3 cups
- Salt 1/2 tsp
- Cornmeal 1 tbsp.

For the Toppings

- Roasted pumpkin cubes 1 cup
- Roasted bell pepper 2 cuts in thin stripes
- Lacinato kale leaves 5 chopped
- Lightly toasted walnuts 1/4 cup
- Pickled onion rings 5-6
- Honey 1 tsp
- Tomato passata 2 tbsp.
- Minced garlic cloves 2
- Extra virgin olive oil 2 tsp
- Pomegranate 1/2 seeds

Instructions

- Water, sugar, and yeast are mixed in a bowl; the yeast should dissolve after ten minutes.
- In a large mixing basin, combine the salt and flour, add the yeast mixture, drizzle in the olive oil, and whisk with a fork.
- When an elastic dough develops, transfer the ingredients to a floured surface and knead for approximately five minutes. Add one more tablespoon of flour if the mixture is too wet.
- The dough should be placed on a dish, covered with a cloth, and let to rise for 30 minutes at room temperature.
- Turn the oven's temperature up to 200 degrees.
- Pizza dough should be shaped into an oval or narrow circular.
- Place the cornmeal over the pizza dough on a cookie sheet covered with bakery release paper.
- Spread the passata thinly on top of the pizza crust before adding the minced kale, pumpkin, and garlic.
- After baking for fifteen minutes, remove from oven and top with pomegranate seeds,

pickled onion, and walnuts.

- Serve heated after adding honey.

Nutrition Facts Per Serving: fat 17 g | Carbohydrate 36 g | Calories 294 | Protein 21 g

23. Spicy Kimchi Tofu Stew

Prep time: 15 mins, Cook time: 20 min, Servings: 6

Ingredients

- Kosher salt
- Silken tofu 1, 16-oz package, cut into 1" pieces
- Vegetable oil 1 tbsp
- Cabbage kimchi gently squeezed 4 cups, chopped, + 1 cup liquid
- Gochujang 2 tbsp
- Scallions 8, cut into 1" pieces
- Reduced-sodium soy sauce 2 tbsp.
- Toasted sesame oil 1 tbsp.
- Black pepper freshly ground
- Toasted sesame seeds 2 tbsp.

Instructions

- Bring a big pot of salted water to a rolling boil. Tofu should be firm and puffy after four minutes of cooking, so turn the heat down to low and gently add the tofu. Transfer the tofu to a medium bowl using a slotted spoon.

- Heat the vegetable oil in a big, heavy saucepan to a medium-high temperature. Gochujang and kimchi should be cooked for 5 to 8 minutes while often stirring before browning. Combine the liquid kimchi with eight cups of water in a large mixing basin. Bring to a low simmer, lower the heat, and cook the kimchi for 35 to 40 minutes until it is smooth and translucent.

- Tofu, soy sauce, and scallions should all be combined in a small pot. The tofu should be heated gently for 20 to 25 minutes or until it has absorbed all the flavors. Add salt and pepper, then pour in the sesame oil. Place the stew in the bowls, then sprinkle sesame seeds on top.

Nutrition Facts Per Serving: fat 19 g | Carbohydrate 48 g | Calories 391 | Protein 23 g

24. Alkaline Chili non-Carne

Prep time: 20 mins, Cook time: 20 min, Servings: 2

Ingredients

- 1 tbsp of olive oil
- 1 onion (chopped)
- 1 crushed garlic clove
- 1 can of chopped tomatoes
- 2 tbsp of tomato puree
- 1 red chili, thinly sliced,
- 1/2 tsp of ground cumin
- 1/2 tsp of ground coriander Bragg Liquid Aminos
- 1/2 veg stock (yeast-free) cube
- Himalayan Salt & black pepper (freshly ground)
- 200g can of red kidney drained beans
- 1 head of chopped broccoli,
- 1 handful of spinach
- Lime wedges to serve

Instructions

- Cook the garlic and onion until they are soft in 50 ml of simmering water or stock in a large, heavy pot.
- Cumin, Bragg Liquid Aminos sauce, powdered coriander, and the crushed stock cube should all be added to the mixture along with the tomato puree, diced tomatoes, and cumin. To thoroughly blend, stir.

- Salt and pepper to taste should be used liberally. Cook the mixture for about 20 minutes, occasionally stirring with a wooden spoon, at a moderate simmer, until it is rich and thickened.

- Include kidney beans and fresh coriander. Before turning off the heat and adding flavorings to taste, simmer under cover for an additional 8 minutes.

- After cooling, add fresh broccoli, spinach, raw and diced, and a little olive oil.

- This recipe pairs wonderfully with lime wedges, rice, guacamole, and a large green salad.

Nutrition Facts Per Serving: Calories 407|fat 11 g | Carbohydrate 42 g| Protein 18 g

25. Tomato Pie with Honey

Prep time: 5 mins, Cook time: 30 min, Servings: 2

Ingredients

For the crust

- Whole wheat flour 2 cups
- Warm water 1/2 cup
- Extra virgin olive oil 2 tbsp.
- Active dry yeast 1/2 tsp
- Granulated sugar 1 tsp
- Salt 1/4 tsp
- To garnish Nigella seeds, 2 tsp
- For the filling
- Tomato mixes 1 &1/2 lb. about 700 g
- Garlic clove 5 unpeeled crushed
- Dijon mustard with seeds 1 tbsp.
- Dried oregano 1 tsp
- Basil leaves plus extra

- Toasted pine nuts 1 tbsp.
- Olive oil extra virgin 2 tsp
- Apple cider vinegar 2 tsp

Instructions

- Set the oven to 175 Celsius for preheating.
- Mix flour, yeast, sugar, and salt in a large mixing basin. To create a dough, mix in the water and olive oil.
- The dough should be kneaded for two to three minutes before being shaped into a 14-inch-diameter thin circle.
- Add two garlic cloves, two basil leaves, and half of the crumbled feta to the circular surface of the dough after spreading the mustard over it.
- Leave a 1-inch border around the edge and cover with tomato slices for seasoning. For a good design, experiment with color and proportion.
- Add the feta, basil, and any leftover garlic cloves to the mixture. Drizzle with olive oil and apple cider vinegar.
- Fold the empty side of the dough over the filling to form a circle for the pie.
- After 40 minutes of cooking, remove from the heat and set aside for 10 minutes before serving.
- Serve warm or chilled and toss with fresh basil and toasted pine nuts. On top, drizzle honey.

Nutrition Facts Per Serving: fat 12 g | Carbohydrate 34 g | Calories 346 | Protein 19 g

26. Black Bean Quinoa Burger with Activated Charcoal Bun

Prep time: 20 mins, Cook time: 25 min, Servings: 2

Ingredients

Patties

- Drained cooked black beans 1 can
- Cooked quinoa 1/2 cup

- Sweet potato 1/2 peeled & grated
- Yellow onion 1 small finely diced
- Minced garlic cloves 4
- Ground cumin 1/2 tsp
- Red chili flakes 1 tsp
- Toasted sesame 2 tsp
- Fresh parsley chopped 1 small bunch
- Sea salt 1/4 tsp
- Drizzle Olive oil

Black bun

- Whole wheat flour 1 cup
- Baking soda 2 tsp
- Apple cider vinegar 1 tbsp.
- Activated charcoal 2 tsp
- Warm almond milk 1/2 cup
- Sea salt
- To decorate Nigella seeds

Instructions

- Turn the oven's temperature up to 200 degrees.
- Combine the flour, salt, charcoal, and bicarbonate of soda in a medium mixing basin.
- Pour the warm almond milk gradually while swirling regularly to create a thick batter.
- Prepare a baking sheet with parchment paper and evenly scoop the mixture to create 2 circular buns.
- Sprinkle with Nigella seeds, drizzle with olive oil, and bake for 20 minutes. Take it out of the oven, then keep it warm by covering it with a fresh towel.

- Take it out of the oven, cover it with a fresh towel, and set it in a warm location.
- Please cook the patties while the buns are baked.
- With a fork, mash the black beans in a large mixing dish to create a lumpy mixture.
- In a mixing bowl, incorporate the remaining ingredients by blending them.
- On the baking sheet, shape the mixture into little patties, bake for 15 minutes, flip them over and bake for an additional 10 minutes.
- To 175 degrees Celsius, reduce the oven's setting.
- 15 minutes of baking, followed by 10 more minutes of roasting after flipping.
- After taking the burger out of the oven, serve it right away.

Nutrition Facts Per Serving: fat 9 g | Carbohydrate 32 g | Calories 317 | Protein 14 g

27. Lentil Pasta with Kale and Marinara Sauce

Prep time: 5 mins, Cook time: 10 min, Servings: 6

Ingredients

- Red lentil pasta1/2 pack dry pasta about 1 cup
- Yellow onion 1 finely diced
- Minced garlic cloves 4
- Kale leaves fresh chopped 1 cup
- diced tomatoes 1 can
- Purified water 1/2 cup
- Sea salt 1/4 tsp
- Balsamic vinegar 1 tsp
- Extra virgin olive oil 1 tbsp.
- Brown sugar 1 tsp
- Black pepper Freshly ground
- Basil leaves chopped

- Hemp hearts 1 tbsp.
- Cherry tomatoes quartered 1 cup
- Toasted pine nuts 1 tbsp.
- Nutritional yeast 1 tbsp.
- To garnish, Fresh mint leaves

Instructions

- Olive oil should be heated in a cast-iron skillet before adding the onion and garlic.
- Over medium heat, cook the onion until it is translucent, about 2/3 of a minute.
- In a medium saucepan, combine the salt, vinegar, sugar, tomatoes, basil, and heat to a boil over medium-high heat.
- For ten to fifteen minutes, bring to a boil while covered. Prepare the lentil spaghetti as directed on the packet in the meanwhile. Five minutes before they are done, add the kale leaves.
- As directed on the packaging, prepare the lentil pasta. The kale leaves should be ready in about 5 minutes after being added.
- Kale and pasta should be drained and kept aside. The pan sauce should incorporate hemp, nutritional yeast, and pine nuts.
- Put the mixture into serving glasses on a plate. Add fresh mint leaves to the dish before serving.

Nutrition Facts Per Serving: fat 26 g | Carbohydrate 47 g | Calories 372 | Protein 12 g

28. Joseph's Best Easy Bacon Recipe

Prep Time: 5 mins, Cook Time: 15 mins, Serving: 6

Ingredients

- 1 package of thick bacon cut

Instructions

- A baking sheet should have two sheets of Al foil covering the whole surface area. On a baking sheet coated with parchment, arrange the bacon in a single layer about half an inch apart. To hasten the cooking process, put the pan in a cold oven. Set the oven temperature to 425 degrees Fahrenheit (220 deg C). 14 minutes is the recommended cooking time for bacon. Place the roasted bacon on trays lined with paper towels. Give the bacon five minutes to cool down and crisp up.

Nutrition Facts Per Serving: fat 10 g | Carbohydrate 34 g | Calories 334 | Protein 9 g

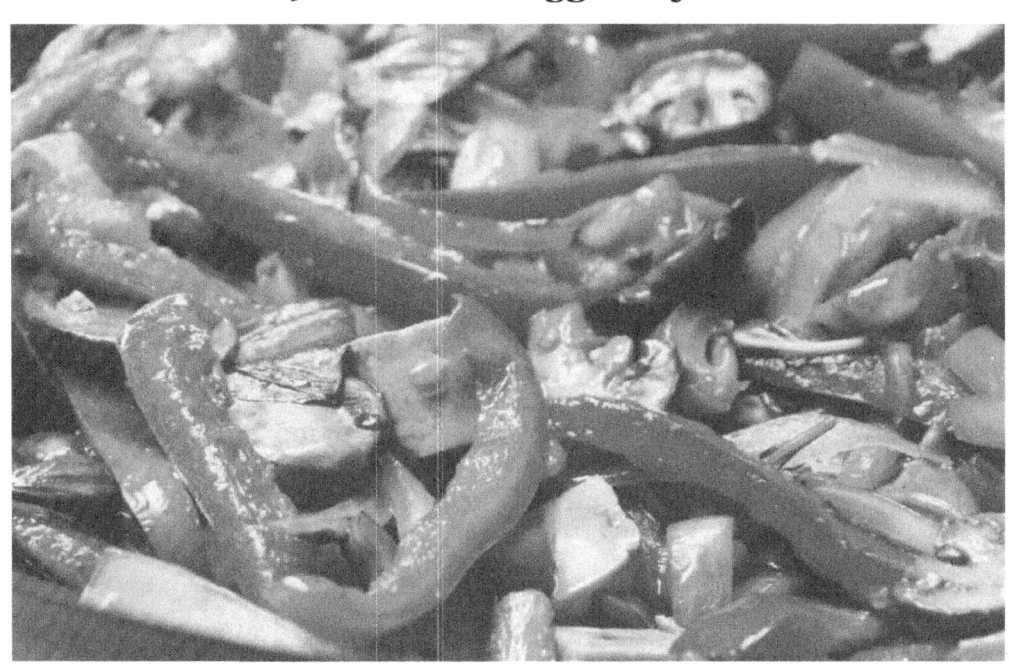

29. Alkaline Veggie Fajitas

Prep time: 20 mins, Cook time: 20 min, Servings: 2

Ingredients

- Tortillas, Wheat-free
- 1 avocado
- Handful spinach
- Broccoli florets
- 1 carrot, grated
- Lettuce leaves
- Paprika
- Pine nuts

- Olive oil
- Red onion
- Tomato
- Coriander

Optional:

- Half a tin of kidney beans
- Half a block of firm tofu

Instructions

- To make salsa, finely slice the tomato and red onion and blend them with olive oil.
- Finely chopped broccoli is cooked gently. Avocado and salsa should be combined, then spread over the wrap.
- In a pan, gently warm the kidney beans and, if desired, mash them.
- Add shredded carrots, pine nuts, herbs, spices, and optional kidney beans to the wrap to create a filling.

Nutrition Facts Per Serving: Calories 367|fat 15 g | Carbohydrate 39 g| Protein 11 g

30. Aubergine & Chickpeas Balti

Prep time: 10 mins, Cook time: 20 min, Servings: 2

Ingredients

- 2 tbsp of coconut oil
- 1 onion, finely sliced
- 1/2 tsp of cumin seeds
- 1 potato
- 1 aubergine
- 1 tin of chickpeas
- 1 tsp of ground coriander

- 1/2 tsp of ground cumin
- 1/4 tsp of turmeric
- Fresh coriander

Instructions

- The cumin seeds and onions should be browned for two minutes in medium-high heat coconut oil.
- The remaining potato slices, chickpeas, aubergine, ground coriander, turmeric, and cumin should then be added. After three more minutes of cooking, turn off the heat.
- You can now make the sauce. Before adding the chopped tomatoes, turmeric, and other spices and savories, immediately add the garlic, onion, ginger, and cloves to the pan and fry for 60 seconds. Increase the amount of coconut oil in the pan. Allow things to develop during the next three minutes.
- In a hand mixer, mash the sauces together roughly (or large blender). Add the vegetables, coriander, water, and any more salt or pepper to taste before mixing everything.
- You need to cook for 20 minutes to be ready. Garnish with fresh coriander and serve with brown rice!

Nutrition Facts Per Serving: Calories 489|fat 7 g | Carbohydrate 41 g| Protein 12 g

31. Roasted cauliflower, fennel, and ginger soup

Prep Time: 3 mins, Cook Time: 20 Mins, Serving: 3

Ingredients

- 1 quartered red onion
- 4 cloves garlic
- ½ large cauliflower head
- 2 chopped & cored fennel bulbs
- 500 g choice stock
- 3 tbsp hummus

- 1 Tbsp Gut Blend Golden
- 1 tsp leaves of sage
- fennel seeds pinch
- 2 tbsp tamari wheat-free
- 2 tbs lemon fresh
- 1 peeled knob of ginger

Instructions

- Turn the oven's temperature up to 200 degrees. Combine the red onion, fennel, and cauliflower on a baking sheet. Until crispy, bake for 30 to 35 minutes.
- Take it out of the oven, then incorporate it with the remaining ingredients. Blend until frothy and smooth for one or two minutes. Put a pot with a thick bottom on the stove. Let flavors meld for the rest of the cooking process on low heat.
- To taste, add salt and pepper to the food. Before serving hot food, give it some time to cool. Fronds of fennel may be used as a garnish.

Nutrition Facts Per Serving: fat 19 g | Carbohydrate 45 g | Calories 357 | Protein 15 g

32. Easy Kielbasa Skillet Dinner

Prep Time: 20 mins, Cook Time: 35 mins, Serving: 4

Ingredients

- ½ chopped onion
- 1 package sliced kielbasa sausage
- cooking spray
- ½ cut head broccoli
- 3 peeled & sliced potatoes
- salt & black pepper ground

Instructions

- Lightly oil an 8-inch skillet and preheat it over medium heat. For five minutes, stir the onion in the oil in a big skillet over medium heat until transparent. Cook the kielbasa for a further 5 minutes, turning often.

- Before incorporating the potatoes and broccoli, season the sausage mixture with salt and pepper. Broccoli will be tender after 15 minutes of uncovered simmering. Cook the veggies for 10 to 15 minutes, stirring periodically, or until they can easily be penetrated with a fork.

Nutrition Facts Per Serving: fat 23 g | Carbohydrate 35 g | Calories 392 | Protein 18 g

33. Easy Dinner Hash

Prep Time: 15 mins, Cook Time: 20 mins, Serving: 2

Ingredients

- 1 tbsp oil vegetable
- 8 oz sausage bulk Italian
- 1 peeled & diced potato
- ¼ chopped onion
- 1 cup mixed vegetables frozen
- to taste salt & pepper

Instructions

- An 8-inch skillet should be lightly oiled and heated over medium heat. Over medium heat, sauté the onion in the oil for 5 minutes, turning periodically, until translucent. Cook the kielbasa for 5 minutes, often turning or until it is lightly browned.

- Add pepper and salt to the sausage mixture before adding the broccoli and potatoes—Cook broccoli for 15 minutes under a covered pot of water. Cook for 10-15 minutes, stirring occasionally, or until the vegetables are tender when poked with a fork.

Nutrition Facts Per Serving: fat 26 g | Carbohydrate 28 g | Calories 422 | Protein 34 g

34. Classic Carrot & Coriander Soup

Prep time: 15 mins, Cook time: 15 min, Servings: 2

Ingredients

- Coconut Oil
- 1 chopped onion
- 2 chopped garlic cloves
- 4 carrots, peeled & chopped
- 400ml of vegetable stock (yeast free)
- 3 tbsp of chopped coriander
- Celtic sea salt
- Black pepper, freshly ground

Instructions

- The onions and garlic should be softened by gently sautéed in coconut oil. It lacks flavor but has a coconutty, tropical fragrance. Maintain a low heat while sautéing the onion until it is soft but not mushy. It would be best if you didn't let the garlic burn.
- Cooking the carrots for a further 3–4 minutes will soften them.
- Stir in the veggies and boil the mixture. After boiling, carrots need to be cooked until they're fork-tender. Don't overcook your meal to maintain nutritional value.
- The last step is to add the coriander and salt, and pepper. Pour into a blender and mix until the required texture is achieved.
- If you want spiciness, you may throw in a touch of cayenne pepper or a dash of ginger.

Nutrition Facts Per Serving: Calories 493|fat 16 g | Carbohydrate 34 g| Protein 25 g

35. Hobo Dinner

Prep Time: 15 mins, Cook Time: 1 hour, Serving: 4

Ingredients

- 5 peeled potatoes
- 4 peeled & sliced lengthwise large carrots
- 1 peeled & sliced in rings onion
- to taste salt
- to taste black pepper ground
- to taste garlic salt

Instructions

- Turn the oven's temperature to 400 degrees (200 degrees C). A baking pan should be lined with aluminum foil.
- Create patties, then cook them in a skillet over medium heat. Place the potatoes, then the carrots, and then the onion rings on the bottom layer. Add kosher salt, fresh cracked pepper, and garlic salt to taste.
- Seal the edges after wrapping the aluminum foil. Depending on how done it is, it makes for an hour.

Nutrition Facts Per Serving: fat 14 g | Carbohydrate 56 g | Calories 351 | Protein 23 g

36. New Year's Day Dinner

Prep Time: 25 mins, Cook Time: 35 mins, Serving: 4

Ingredients

- 1 tbsp of butter
- ½ shredded head of cabbage
- 1 diced onion
- ½ tsp seeds caraway
- to taste, salt & black pepper ground

- 1 & ½ cups divided broth
- 1 diced bell pepper red
- 1 diced bell pepper green

Instructions

- Cook and stir in heated vegetable oil in a medium pan over medium heat for approximately 10 minutes or until browned. Put the aside after adding it to a large mixing bowl. Butter should be melted in a large pan over medium heat. Sauté and toss the cabbage for 5 minutes or until it has wilted. After adding the onion to the cabbage, cook it for approximately 5 minutes, often turning.

- In addition to adding half a cup of broth stock, season to taste with salt, caraway seeds, and black pepper. After the broth almost evaporates, turn the heat to moderate and whisk in the last cup of liquid. Add the green and red bell peppers, cover the pan and simmer for 10 minutes or until the peppers soften.

Nutrition Facts Per Serving: fat 13 g | Carbohydrate 18 g | Calories 278 | Protein 23 g

37. Autumn Tomato & Avocado Warmer

Prep time: 20 mins, Cook time: 10 min, Servings: 2

Ingredients

- 5 ripe tomatoes
- 1 ripe avocado
- 1 spring onion
- 1/4 cup of almonds
- 1 cup of broth from
- Vegetable bouillon, Swiss
- 1/4 tsp. of dill seed
- Dash cayenne Chilli
- Sea salt with black pepper for taste

Instructions

- Blend the other ingredients (apart from the tomato) in a blender.
- You may quickly heat soup in a pot to make it hot or cold. The soup is still uncooked even after it has been reheated to the point that sticking your finger in it doesn't hurt.
- Slice the remaining tomato and sprinkle it on top as a garnish.

Nutrition Facts Per Serving: Calories 465|fat 9.3 g | Carbohydrate 52 g| Protein 18.1 g

38. Alkaline Gazpacho

Prep time: 15 mins, Cook time: 10 min, Servings: 2

Ingredients

- 500 ml juiced tomatoes
- 1 cucumber, juiced
- 1/4 pepper
- 1 stick celery
- 1/2 clove garlic
- basils leave
- Olive oil

Instructions

- Juice the cucumbers and tomatoes, then combine the results.
- Chopped celery, peppers, and garlic are added to the soup.
- Mix thoroughly after adding the basil and oil. You may adjust the seasoning to your liking.
- The ratio of tomato and cucumber will determine whether the sauce is thicker or thinner. Red pepper will enhance taste and sweetness.

Nutrition Facts Per Serving: Calories 375|fat 15 g | Carbohydrate 48 g| Protein 14 g

39. Chopped Veggie Grain Bowls with Turmeric Dressing

Prep time: 10 mins, Cook time: 10 mins, Servings: 4

Ingredients:

- 2 packages of cooked quinoa
- 1 container of veggie mix, chopped
- 1 can of chickpeas, rinsed
- 1/2 cup of dressing of turmeric salad

Instructions

- Cook the quinoa. Let the transfer utterly cool in a shallow dish before combining the bowls.
- For the vegetable mixture, four single serving covered containers should be used. Each of the four pizzas must have a quarter of quinoa and a quarter of chickpeas. After filling and closing the containers, freeze them for four days.
- Transfer 2 tablespoons of salad dressing into each 4 little, sealed containers, and then freeze for 4 days.
- The dressing should be poured into each bowl just before serving.

Nutrition Facts Per Serving: Calories 306 | fat 8 g | Carbohydrates 48 g | Protein 12 g

40. Alkaline Raw Soup

Prep time: 10 mins, Cook time: 10 min, Servings: 2

Ingredients

- 1 avocado
- 2 onions
- 1/2 green pepper
- 1 cucumber
- 2 handfuls spinach
- 1/2 clove garlic
- Bragg Liquid Aminos for taste

- 100ml vegetable Bouillon
- 1 lemon Juice

Instructions

- Other ingredients may be added, and the procedure may be repeated after the stock and avocado have been combined into a light paste.

Nutrition Facts Per Serving: Calories 368|fat 12 g | Carbohydrate 39 g| Protein 16 g

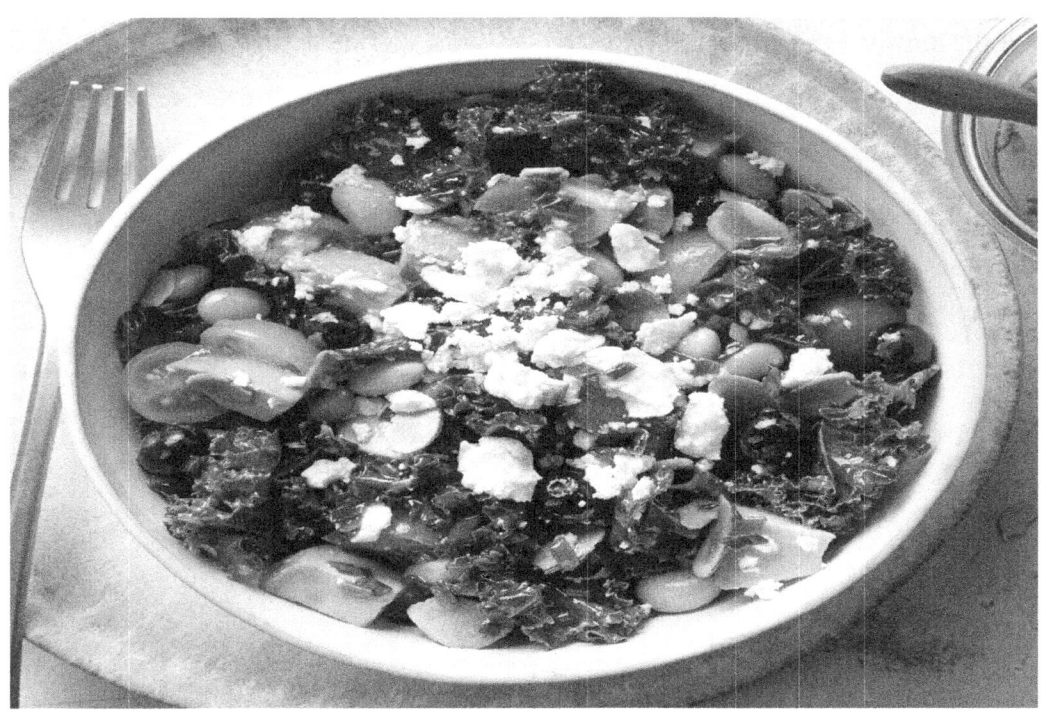

41. Kale & Avocado Salad with Blueberries & Edamame

Prep time: 20 mins, Cook time: 20 mins, Servings: 4

Ingredients

- 6 cups of curly kale
- 1 avocado
- 1 cup of blueberries
- 1 cup of cherry tomatoes, halved yellow
- 1 cup of shelled edamame, cooked
- ¼ cup of sliced almonds

- ¼ cup of olive oil
- 3 tbsp. of lemon juice
- 1 tbsp of minced chives
- 1 ½ tsp. of honey
- 1 tsp of Dijon mustard
- 1 tsp of salt

Instructions

- Use your hands to gently massage the kale leaves in a big bowl to make them softer. Tomatoes, blueberries, and avocado are other acceptable additions.
- To create the dressing, combine all the ingredients in a small container and securely screw the lid. Whether you're whisking or shaking, do it thoroughly.
- After the vinaigrette has been spread over the salad, toss it.

Nutrition Facts Per Serving: Calories 368 | fat 29 g | Carbohydrates 21 g | Protein 10 g

42. Alkaline Tom Yum Soup

Prep time: 20 mins, Cook time: 10 min, Servings: 2

Ingredients

- Lemongrass 1 stick
- 1-2 red chilies
- Half brown onion (large chunks)
- Galangal (two small strips)
- Fresh ginger, the same amount
- 2 kefir lime leaves
- Handful of coriander
- Garlic 2 cloves
- 2 tomatoes, quartered

- 600ml vegetable stock
- Soy Sauce or Bragg Liquid Aminos (Bragg is more alkaline)
- Handful of beansprouts
- Cubed tofu in any quantity you choose.

Instructions

- Make all the tastes first. Ginger and galangal should be cut into thin strips, the chili stem should be removed, the chili should not be chopped, and the lemongrass should be cut into 1.5-inch pieces and beaten flat once more.
- Slice all the lime leaves in half and crush the garlic. You must be drooling right about now just thinking about these mouthwatering tastes.
- Bring the liquid and onion to a boil in the saucepan after that. Add the tofu when the sauce has bubbled and come to a boil. Add the tomato and, if wanted, the coriander and beansprouts after two minutes. Serve the meal soon away after removing it from the heat.
- The soup must be delicious and heated. If you want to make it a bit sweeter and are alright with it not being completely alkaline, add a pinch of brown sugar or palm sugar. Pepper and salt to taste. Enjoy!

Nutrition Facts Per Serving: Calories 379|fat 16.8 g | Carbohydrate 49 g| Protein 9 g

Chapter 5: Snacks and Appetizers

During your holidays when you feel hunger pang sensations snacks & appetizers can fulfil your needs. Here you will find great diversity of snacks and appetizers recipes.

1. Fruit Race Cars for Kids

Prep Time: 10 mins, Cook Time: 0 mins, Serving: 2

Ingredients

- Apples
- Knife
- Cutting board
- Seedless grapes
- Rounded toothpicks

Instructions

- Cleaning and prepping your fruit should come first. To get rid of waxy buildup, rinse with water and then use a bicarbonate soda and salt solution. Rinsing and drying should be done again.
- The apple should be cut into thirds twice. There is enough nourishment in one apple to feed 12 people.
- Make a clean cut around the apple to get the core and seeds out.
- Transversely insert two toothpicks into each flat end of the apple wedge.
- Grapes should be placed halfway up toothpicks. The automobile would be more stable if the grapes were larger.

Nutrition Facts Per Serving: fat 11 g | Carbohydrate 43 g | Calories 318 | Protein 10 g

2. Hot garlic ginger Lemonade

Prep time: 10 mins, Cook time: 30 mins, Servings: 2

Ingredients

- Fresh garlic cloves3 to 4 chopped, minced or grated
- Fresh ginger1 tsp - peel, then mince or grate
- Boiling filtered water4 cups
- Organic lemon1, juiced
- bgrade2 tbsp

Instructions

- Peeling and cutting have been done to prepare the ginger and garlic.
- Bring the water to a boil in a saucepan or tea kettle.
- Garlic cloves, astragalus root, and ginger root are combined in a quart-sized mason jar or heatproof glass jar. Boiling water should be added to a saucepan halfway. Continue carefully into the heatproof glass or Mason jar. Cover and steep for about 30 minutes.
- Use a sieve with a small hole to pour into a fresh mason jar or glass container.
- The ginger-garlic combination should be sweetened with your preferred sweetener and one lemon juice.
- Serve right now or keep in the fridge for later. Just before serving, reheat it.

Nutrition Facts Per Serving: Calories 324 | fat 12 g | Carbohydrates 39 g | Protein 28 g

3. The Ginger Shot That Will Keep Cold and Flu Away

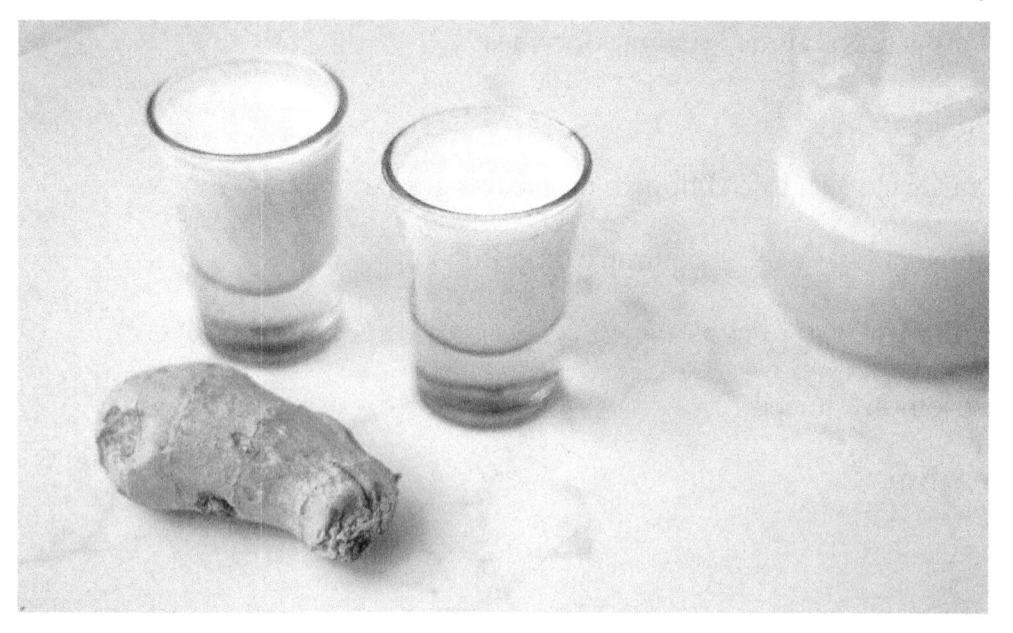

Prep time: 20 mins, Cook time: 0 mins, Servings: 1

Ingredients

- Juicy lemons 2 big
- Honey 2-3 tbsp
- Ginger 25 grams

Instructions

- Start pressing the lemon(s) to release the juice and drain it. Even the pulp may be saved, but it would be too heavy to drink since it contains little pieces of ginger.
- Honey and lemon juice should be combined in a mixer.
- Add the ginger to the blender once it has been cut into tiny pieces.
- For 30 to 60 seconds, combine everything. Given that the honey is thick, we want it to be well incorporated. Ginger cannot be made into a paste or anything similar due to its gritty nature.

Nutrition Facts Per Serving: Calories 395 | fat 7 g | Carbohydrates 32 g | Protein 24 g

4. Turmeric, ginger, & lemon shots

Prep time: 10 mins, Cook time: 0 mins, Servings: 1

Ingredients

- Turmeric root ~7 oz (large handful)
- Lemons 3 to 4, rind removed
- Ginger root ~6 oz chopped
- Sweet apple 1, quartered
- Black pepper (Pinch)

Instructions

- Blend the ingredients in a blender, then pass the pulp through a strainer lined with cloth.
- To preserve the juice, put it in the bottles and one big jar with ice cube trays.
- Pour two ounces into a cup to serve, then top with black pepper. Now take a seat and unwind.

Nutrition Facts Per Serving: Calories 299 | fat 4 g | Carbohydrates 28 g | Protein 20 g

5. Ginger Lemon Immune Boosting Shots

Prep time: 07 mins, Cook time: 0 mins, Servings: 1

Ingredients

- Ginger root 450 gr
- Lemons 6
- Honey1 tsp or agave/maple
- Cayenne pepper 1/8 tsp

Instructions

- Start by cleaning the ginger root with a brush and water. It must be peeled and cut into tiny pieces to fit through the juicer.
- The ginger should then be juiced first.

- Ensure the output is accurate and the lemons are sufficiently juiced if the ginger has been juiced. Peel and white rind may go through the juicer if they are removed. Alternately, you may weigh the lemon juice and ginger juice in a 1:1 ratio.

- Ginger and lemon juice should be combined.

- Mix the honey, cayenne, agave, and maple syrup in a large bowl.

- After splitting into 60 mL (shot-sized) portions, refrigerate for up to a week. Cayenne pepper will spill out, so give the shot bottle a good shake before taking a sip.

- You can also chill the juice in ice cubes and add it to beverages and smoothies if necessary.

Nutrition Facts Per Serving: Calories 408 | fat 7 g | Carbohydrates 48 g | Protein 35 g

6. Pineapple turmeric sauerkraut and gut shots

Prep time: 20 mins, Cook time: 0 mins, Servings: 3

Ingredients

- Cabbage head 1 (shredded)
- Pineapple ½ (chopped)
- Ground turmeric 1 tbsp
- Fresh ginger 1 tbsp (grated)
- Brine
- Sea salt 1 tbsp
- Purified water 4 cups

Instructions

- Place the cabbage in a mixing basin and mandolin or finely chop it. Put everything into a large mixing bowl.

- Place the pineapple on the plate with the cabbage after chopping it into tiny pieces.

- Sea salt and chopped ginger should be added to the mixing bowl.

- Five minutes or until the combination decomposes and becomes mushy should be spent massaging the cabbage mixture with your hands.

- Give it 15 minutes to rest in the bowl.
- The cabbage would be incredibly moist and tender after fifteen minutes. Press it now, and juice will start to stream out.
- The cabbage should be supplemented with curcumin. You may either mix it with your hands or a spoon. Use a spoon if you don't want your hands and fingernails to become orange from the curcumin.
- Making the brine and placing it in the jars for the gut shots will come first.
- One cup of salt and boiling water will form the brine. When the salt has dissolved, drain the extra water, and add the apple cider vinegar.
- After adding the brine to the mason jars, leave an inch of room at the top.
- In a saucepan, mix the cabbage and brine by stirring.
- The jar should have a light cover to let gas escape during fermentation.
- Place in a cool, shaded area on the counter for 4 to 7 days.
- The sauerkraut will bubble up and get murky during fermentation. Take any scum that emerges with a spoon.
- Shake the mason jar for a day or two to ensure the cabbage is well buried in the brine.
- Serve cooled after placing in the fridge.

Nutrition Facts Per Serving: Calories 316 | fat 18 g | Carbohydrates 38 g | Protein 29 g

7. How to make probiotic-rich water kefir

Prep time: 10 mins, Cook time: 0 mins, Servings: 1

Ingredients

- Brown Sugar ¼ Cup
- Liquid Minerals ½ cap (optional)
- Quart Water

Instructions

- Spring water should be poured into the mason jar until it is complete. Then, add the minerals and brown sugar, and mix to combine.

- After adding the kefir grains, add the last of the water. Place the cover in place and let it be there for two days.

- The water kefir should be filtered into mason jars or plastic pitchers using a wooden strainer or plastic and kept in the fridge. To make a bigger batch, repeat this recipe.

- Drink it straight up or combine it with your preferred juice.

Nutrition Facts Per Serving: Calories 359 | fat 9 g | Carbohydrates 36 g | Protein 22 g

8. Vanilla bean and honey kefir panna cotta

Prep time: 15 mins, Cook time: 0 mins, Servings: 1

Ingredients

- Plain milk kefir 2 cups
- Honey 1 tbsp
- Hot water ¼ cup of
- Chopped strawberries 3 cups

Instructions

- Combine the kefir, honey, and vanilla in a saucepan.
- Warm the kefir slowly by lowering the heat. The only thing left to do is warm it up. The beneficial bacteria could be eliminated if the temperature increases more.
- Continue stirring once the vanilla and honey have been well combined.
- Put the gelatin powder on a plate, then pour warm water. It must be thoroughly dissolved by mixing.
- Gently stir the gelatin mixture into the hot kefir as you do so.
- Blend everything until it's smooth and creamy.
- After putting it into glasses, refrigerate for several hours or overnight.
- Before serving, sprinkle the Panna Cotta with the finely chopped raspberries.

Nutrition Facts Per Serving: Calories 257 | fat 16 g | Carbohydrates 31 g | Protein 19 g

9. Lemon verbena kombucha

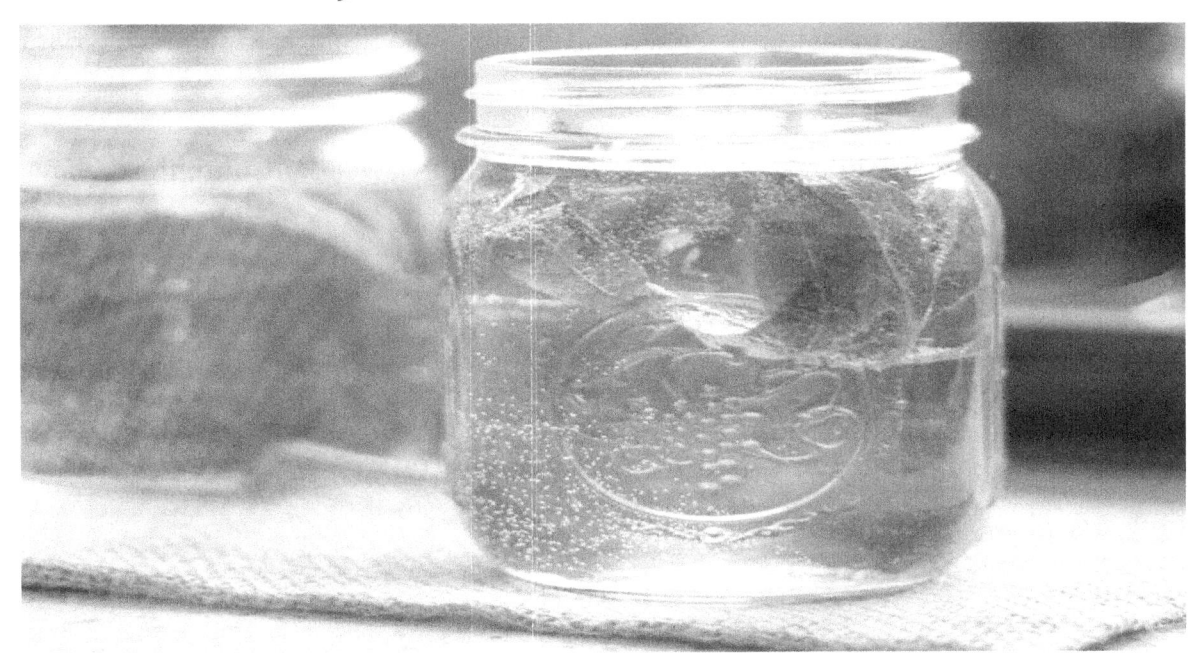

Prep time: 20 mins, Cook time: 0 mins, Servings: 1

Ingredients

- Green tea kombucha ½ gallon
- Fresh lemon verbena leaves 2 cups
- Hot water 1 cup
- Sugar 1 tbsp of

Instructions

- One glass of water should come to a boil.
- Lemon bee brush leaves should be boiled in boiling water for 15 minutes.
- Remove the leaves using a sieve, then stir in some sugar. Mix everything until everything dissolves.
- Wait until the tea is at room temperature.
- Combine the basic kombucha with the chilled lemon verbena tea in a big pitcher.
- Fill the flip-top bottles with kombucha using a funnel.
- Cover the bottles in plastic wrap for three to seven days and keep them somewhere dark

and cold.

- Check one of the bottles after three days; if it is bubbling, put it in the refrigerator. Only serve cold.

- Let it air out for a few more days if it isn't bubbling. Review it daily until the carbonation is complete.

- Serve it cold and keep it in the refrigerator.

Nutrition Facts Per Serving: Calories 323 | fat 16 g | Carbohydrates 28 g | Protein 24 g

10. Ginger beet sauerkraut

Prep time: 20 mins, Cook time: 0 mins, Servings: 2

Ingredients

- Beets grated 3
- Cabbage head 1 shredded
- Ginger peeled 1" and thinly sliced/grated
- Sea salt 1 tbsp

Instructions

- Take three of the outer leaves from the cabbage head. Chop the remaining cabbage using a mandolin or a mixing bowl. Salt the ginger and beets and add them to a big mixing basin.

- With your hands, massage the cabbage mixture until it disintegrates and softens (approximately five mins). After that, kindly let it rest for another fifteen minutes so that it may collapse even more and produce additional juices.

- Push the cabbage all the way down into the juices in the mason jar to cover it entirely. The distance between the jar's highest point and the gap should be 112 inches. Make more brine by mixing one glass of water and one teaspoon of sea salt if there isn't enough to cover the cabbage.

- The cabbage leaves should be rolled up and put in a jar so they may be submerged in the brine. Loosen the lid's screw when fermentation starts to allow gas to escape. Place in a cool, shaded area on a counter for five to seven days. The sauerkraut would bubble up and become cloudy during fermentation. If scum develops, use a spoon to scrape it off.

- Before serving, please take out the folded cabbage leaves and toss them.

Nutrition Facts Per Serving: Calories 269 | fat 13 g | Carbohydrates 24 g | Protein 18 g

11. Jalapeno cilantro sauerkraut

Prep time: 30 mins, Cook time: 0 mins, Servings: 2

Ingredients

- Cabbage head 1 shredded
- Sea salt 1 tbsp of
- Jalapeños 4, seeds removed
- Garlic clove 2
- Cilantro ½ cup
- Onion ½

Instructions

- The cabbage head's top three leaves should be removed and set aside. Chop the remaining cabbage with a knife and place it in a mixing basin or mandolin. Put it into the sizable mixing basin.
- After approximately five minutes of mixing, sprinkle the cabbage with salt and give it a good massage.
- Remove the cabbage from the pan and let it sit for 15 to 20 minutes to let the sea salt drain the liquid and make it soft.
- Next, remove the seeds from the jalapenos, or leave them in for the spicier kraut, and put them in a mixing bowl over medium heat. Use caution while managing the peppers as they may burn and irritate the skin and eyes. When handling this, put on gloves, and wash your hands well afterward.
- In a mixing dish, combine the cilantro, onion, and garlic and pulse until everything is finely chopped.
- Please return to the cabbage and mix and compress it with your hands. When a liquid is squeezed, if any spills appear, it is ready for another motion.

- Whisk in the cabbage before adding it to the jalapeño mixture. Use your hands unless you are wearing gloves; otherwise, use the spoon.

- Put the cabbage into the ball jar and compress it tightly using a gloved or veggie hand. Until it is completely immersed in its liquids, push it down.

- Repeat this procedure until there are about 1 1/2 inches of space between the highest point of the jar and the top of the lid.

- To press the cabbage beneath the brine, fold the leaves and put them in the jar.

- Loosen the lid's screw when fermentation starts to allow gas to escape. Place in a cool, shaded area on the counter for five to seven days. If the ball/mason jar overflows and creates a mess, place a plate under it.

- The sauerkraut would bubble up and become cloudy during fermentation. If scum develops, use a spoon to scrape it clean.

- Before serving, please take out the folded cabbage leaves and toss them.

- It must be stored in the fridge.

Nutrition Facts Per Serving: Calories 297 | fat 11 g | Carbohydrates 41 g | Protein 37 g

12. Homemade Kimchi

Prep time: 1.5 hours, Cook time: 0 mins, Servings: 3

Ingredients

- Napa cabbage 1 lb
- Water 1-2 cups
- Daikon radish 1/2 cup (julienned)
- Carrot 1 (julienned)
- Green onion 3 stalks

Paste

- Chili flakes 1-3 tbsp
- Cloves garlic 2 (grated)

- Ginger 1/2 cube (grated)
- Sugar 1 tbsp

Instructions

- To create more bite-sized pieces, cut the napa cabbage half widthwise. Please don't make the cabbage too tiny since it will shrink as it cooks. Keep the rigid cores for a future soup or discard them after removing them.

- Sliced cabbage and salt should be combined in a big mixing basin, and after 10 minutes, your hands should massage the mixture. The cabbage is starting to fade up and wilt. Place the cabbage on top of the water and let it for an hour. Put a heavy object on top of it to keep it buried.

- Place all ingredients in a blender and process until smooth to create the chili paste. Add one or three tablespoons of chili flakes to make it spicier. Since sugar feeds the bacteria and speeds up fermentation, you may exclude it from the recipe.

- After the cabbage is soaked, rinse it for approximately five minutes in cold water, ensuring all the leaves are clean. Then thoroughly rub the cabbage leaves with the radish, carrot, chili paste, and green onion. Keep your gloves on tightly to prevent hand burn and discoloration.

- Use hot water to thoroughly clean the jar and its lid. Dry it before you fill it. Put as much kimchi as you can into the jar. As soon as you see the water boiling, ensure the contents are at the top of the jar.

- For two to five days, let it ferment at room temperature. You may use a clean spoon to reach into the jar and massage the contents downward if they are dehydrated. Put the leftovers in the refrigerator when you've done eating them.

Nutrition Facts Per Serving: Calories 287 | fat 12 g | Carbohydrates 39 g | Protein 24 g

13. Healthy homemade lemonade (naturally sweetened)

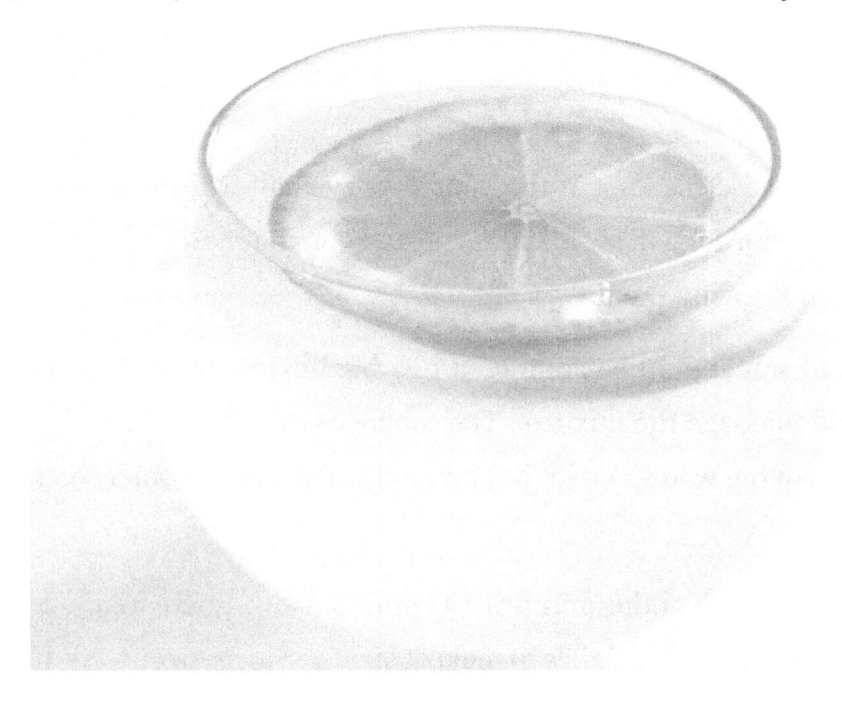

Prep time: 10 mins, Cook time: 0 mins, Servings: 1

Ingredients

- Water 6 cups
- 1/3–1/2 cup light-tasting honey or agave
- Fresh lemon juice 1 cup
- Fruit puree Optional
- Few sprigs of fresh mint/basil Optional

Instructions

- In a saucepan or microwave, warm one glass of water until it is scorchingly hot to the touch (but not simmering).
- The honey should be thoroughly dissolved after being added.
- The honey mixture should be added to the pitcher.
- Lemon juice and water should be added.
- Use water when combining herbs or fruit purée.
- Add more agave/honey purée and fresh herbs as needed. Toss to combine.

- Keep the lemonade in the fridge for at least a week.

Nutrition Facts Per Serving: Calories 357 | fat 14 g | Carbohydrates 42 g | Protein 35 g

14. Avocado and Herb Salad

Prep time: 10 mins, Cook time: 0 mins, Servings: 1

Ingredients

- Ripe firm avocados 2-3
- Lemon 1
- Green onions 3 thinly sliced
- Capers 2 tbsp
- Jalapeño pepper minced 1
- Fresh cilantro rough chopped and stems removed
- Fresh parsley rough chopped and stems removed from the dressing
- Extra virgin olive oil 1/4 cup
- Orange blossom vinegar 3 tbsp
- Clove garlic minced 1
- Salt and black pepper

Instructions

- Slice the avocado thinly, then squeeze some lemon juice over it.
- Put all the ingredients in a large, shallow serving dish, including the capers, green onions, spices, and jalapeño.
- Sprinkle the salad with the dressing after combining the ingredients. Serve right away with freshly crushed coarse black pepper.

Nutrition Facts Per Serving: Calories 357 | fat 8 g | Carbohydrates 46 g | Protein 32 g

15. All-natural tamarind paste

Prep time: 10 mins, Cook time: 01 hour, Servings: 1

Ingredients

- Natural tamarind 250 gr
- Springwater 3 cups

Instructions

- Tamarind should be cleaned. Any skin, unwanted component, or seed should be removed. Boil two cups of water while you wait.
- For 45 to 60 minutes, soak your tamarind in two cups of hot water.
- This should be well blended at high speed until the tamarind is soft. The resulting mixture should be strained using a fine-mesh strainer. Stones, trash, and seeds should all be discarded. Over medium heat, simmer the resultant pulp for about five minutes.
- Store the pasta in airtight containers after it has cooled.

Nutrition Facts Per Serving: Calories 408 | fat 8 g | Carbohydrates 37 g | Protein 28 g

16. Tea Recipe Five Flavored Autumn

Prep time: 10 mins, Cook time: 25 mins, Servings: 1

Ingredients

- Dried astragalus 15 g
- Dried oat straw 10 g
- Dried rose hips de-seeded 10
- Dried dandelion root Roasted 10 g
- Dried cinnamon chips 3 g or cinnamon stick 1 broken into pieces
- Water 4 cups
- Apple juice 1 cup

Instructions

- Water and herbs are combined in a medium pot. Bring to a boil, then cover and simmer for

30 minutes on low heat. Add the apple juice after turning the heat off. Give yourself a five-minute break. Strain. You may choose to consume it hot or cold.

Nutrition Facts Per Serving: Calories 318| fat 14 g | Carbohydrates 46 g | Protein 32 g

17. Psyllium Apple & Lemon Balm Tea

Prep time: 05 mins, Cook time: 0 mins, Servings: 1

Ingredients:

- Apple 1
- Lemon balm tea 1 cup, cooled
- Psyllium husk powder 2 tsp
- True cinnamon ¼ tsp

Instructions:

- Combine all the ingredients, then eat.

Nutrition Facts Per Serving: Calories 267 | fat 7 g | Carbohydrates 29 g | Protein 22 g

18. Immunity-boosting soup

Prep time: 10 mins, Cook time: 0 mins, Servings: 1

Ingredients

- Onion 1/2
- Bell pepper 1
- Mushrooms 1 cup (any kind, except shiitake)
- Grapeseed oil 1 tbsp of
- noodles 1 pack (spelled wild rice, amaranth, etc.)
- Key lime 1
- Zucchini 1
- Cherry tomatoes 1 cup
- Water cups 4

- Herbs
- Cayenne pepper and Sea salt

Instructions

- Noodles should be cooked as directed on the box.
- The onion should be diced up. The onion should be sautéed in hot grapeseed oil until it becomes translucent.
- Cut the bell pepper, cherry tomatoes, and mushrooms into tiny pieces. You may sauté in a pan as well. Once the courgette has been cut, please put it in the pan.
- Mix the sea salt, herbs, pepper, and water in a dish. Over medium heat, bring everything to a gentle simmer. Until it reaches the boiling point, turn the heat down. In a bowl, place the cooked noodles. Give it another 10 minutes to boil.
- Make any topping changes that are required. Add extra herbs and critical lime juice before serving.

Nutrition Facts Per Serving: Calories 312 | fat 11 g | Carbohydrates 38 g | Protein 32 g

19. Nori-burritos

Prep time: 10 mins, Cook time: 0 mins, Servings: 1

Ingredients:

- Ripe avocado 1
- Cucumber (seeded) 450 gr
- Ripe mango 1/2
- Nori seaweed 4 sheets
- Zucchini 1, small
- Amaranth/dandelion greens (handful)
- sprouted hemp seeds (handful)
- Tahini 1 tbs
- Sesame seeds

Instructions:

- The Nori sheet should be placed on a cutting board.
- The nori sheet should have an inch of exposed nori to the right as you layer all the ingredients.
- Using your hands, fold the nori sheet from the edge closest to you up and over the package's contents. Slice into thick pieces, then sprinkle with sesame seeds.

Nutrition Facts Per Serving: Calories 357 | fat 13 g | Carbohydrates 38 g | Protein 27 g

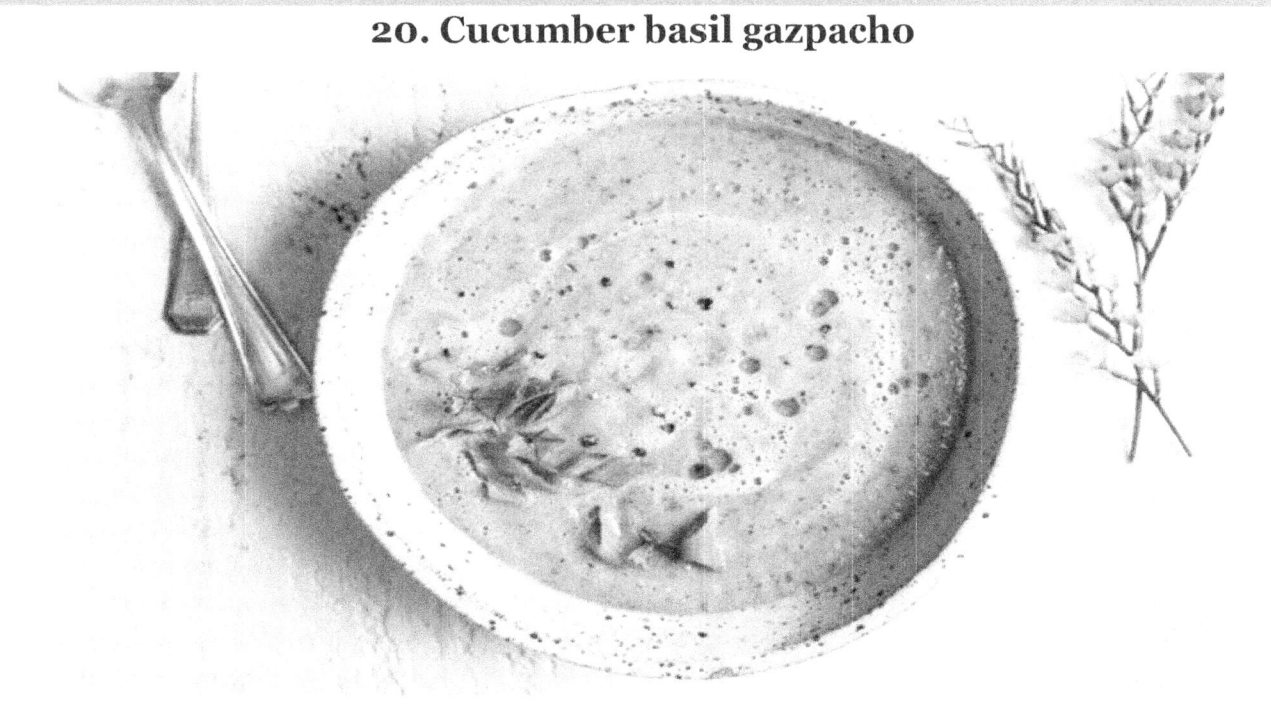

20. Cucumber basil gazpacho

Prep time: 15 mins, Cook time: 0 mins, Servings: 1

Ingredients

- Ripe avocado perfectly 1
- Seeded cucumber 1: skin left; seeds removed
- Handfuls fresh basil 2 small
- Water 2 cups
- Sea salt 1 1/4 tsp of
- 1 key lime juice

Instructions

- Make "gazpacho," this cold soup. To make sure everything is chilly, put it all in the fridge.
- Blend the cooled ingredients till smooth, leaving some green bits behind. To fully cool the soup before serving, place it back in the refrigerator.
- The top is garnished with basil leaves and rings of thinly sliced cucumber.

Nutrition Facts Per Serving: Calories 369 | fat 14 g | Carbohydrates 37 g | Protein 26 g

---

21. Dandelion strawberry salad

Prep time: 05 mins, Cook time: 10 mins, Servings: 1

Ingredients:

- Grapeseed oil 2 tbsp.
- Sliced medium red onion 1
- Strawberries ripe sliced 10
- Essential lime juice 2 tbsp.
- Dandelion greens 4 cups
- Sea salt

Instructions:

- In a 12-inch nonstick frying pan, warm grape seed oil over low heat. Apply a heaping teaspoon of sea salt and some thinly sliced onions. Cook the onions, often turning, until they are smooth, slightly orange, and reduced to about one-third of their initial size.
- Combine the raspberry slices and 1 tsp of key lime juice in a small dish. If preferred, wash the dandelion greens, and cut them into bite-sized pieces. When the onions are almost done, add the remaining lime juice to the pan and simmer for a further minute or two to coat the onions. Take the blame off the onions. Combine the onions, raspberries, and greens in a salad dish with all their juices. Add a little salt to taste.

Nutrition Facts Per Serving: Calories 398 | fat 11 g | Carbohydrates 42 g | Protein 21 g

22. Carrot & Courgetti Stack

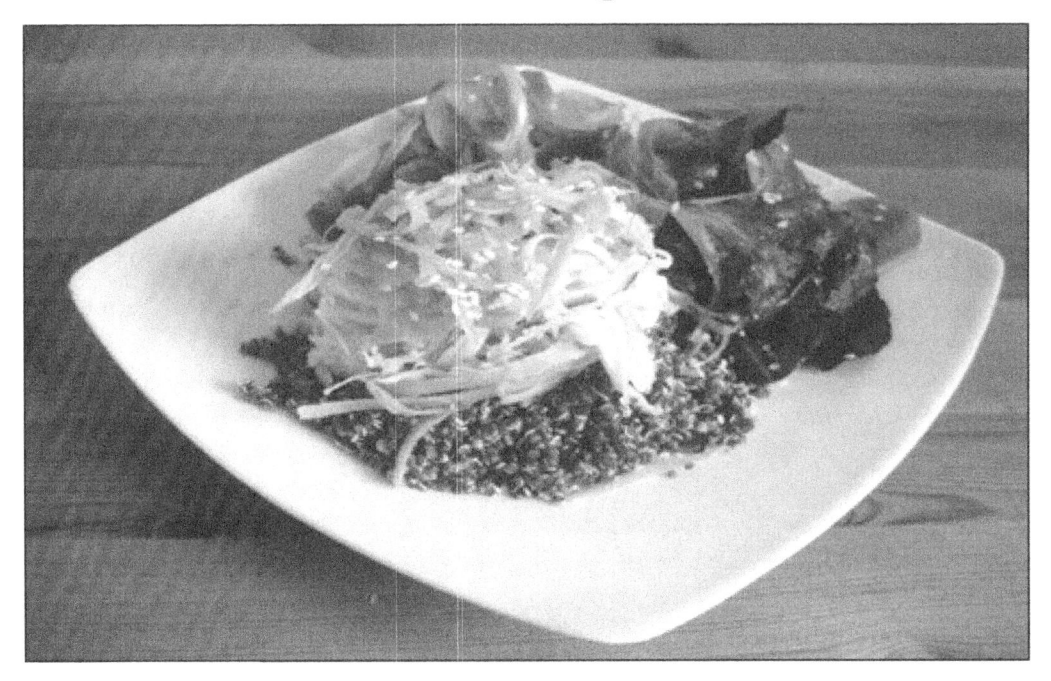

Prep time: 20 mins, Cook time: 10 min, Servings: 2

Ingredients

- 2 serves of quinoa
- Handful leaves of baby spinach
- 1 carrot
- ½ avocado
- 1 courgette
- 1 lime or lemon
- Sesame seeds
- Avocado/Olive oil

Instructions

- Quinoa should be cooked, and a layer of quinoa should be placed on each plate.
- Both the carrot and the courgette should be finely diced before stacking.
- Add spinach, avocado, sesame seeds, lemon juice, and oil.
- To suit your tastes, adjust the seasoning.

Nutrition Facts Per Serving: Calories 336|fat 17 g | Carbohydrate 38 g| Protein 8 g

23. Matcha Green Tea Latte

Prep time: 05 mins, Cook time: 10 mins, Servings: 1

Ingredients

- ¼ cup of boiling water
- 1 tsp of tea powder, matcha
- 1 cup of milk, low-fat
- 1 tsp of honey

Instructions

- Hot water and matcha powder should be combined and mixed until foamy. Bring the milk and honey just to the point of boiling. Milk should be forcefully whisked until frothy. Tea and milk should be combined in a cup after being added.

Nutrition Facts Per Serving: Calories 124 | fat 2 g | Carbohydrates 18 g | Protein 8 g

24. Winter Kale & Quinoa Salad with Avocado

Prep time: 15 mins, Cook time: 35 mins, Servings: 2

Ingredients

- 1 sweet potato
- 2 ½ tsp. of olive oil, divided
- ½ avocado
- 1 tbsp. of lime juice
- 1 clove of garlic, peeled
- ½ tsp of ground cumin
- ⅛ tsp of salt
- ⅛ tsp of ground pepper
- 1-2 tbsp. of water

- 1 cup of cooked quinoa
- ¾ cup of black beans
- 1 ½ cups of chopped baby kale
- 2 tbsp. of pepitas
- 1 scallion

Instructions

- Before you start baking, preheat the oven to 400 °F.
- Spread the sweet potato equally after tossing it with 1 tbsp of oil on a large baking sheet. For 30 minutes, bake. Roast for 25 minutes, stirring about midway through, or until fork tender.
- The remaining 1 1/2 teaspoons of oil should be blended with the other ingredients to form the dressing. Process the mixture until it is completely smooth. Adding 1 tbsp of water may change the consistency as needed.
- Combine kale, black beans, quinoa, and sweet potatoes in a bowl. After drizzling, gently toss with an avocado dressing. On top, sprinkle pepitas and scallions.

Nutrition Facts Per Serving: Calories 439 | fat 20 g | Carbohydrates 54 g | Protein 15 g

25. Spiced Pecans

Prep time: 20 mins, Cook time: 1 hour 20 mins, Servings: 20

Ingredients

- 1 tbsp of water
- 6 tbsp. of superfine sugar
- ½ tsp of kosher salt
- ¼ tsp of ground allspice
- ¼ tsp of ground cloves
- ¼ tsp of ground nutmeg
- Pinch ground cinnamon

- Pinch cayenne pepper
- 4 cups of pecan halves

Instructions

- Before commencing, preheat the oven to 275 °F. A big baking sheet should first be covered with parchment paper.
- Combine all remaining ingredients—aside from the cayenne pepper—in a large mixing dish. The pecans should be well mixed in and coated. To taste, add salt and pepper. Spread the mixture evenly using a spatula on the prepared baking sheet.
- For around 30 minutes, bake. For 30 minutes, bake the nuts while turning the pan from back to front. After that, let it completely cool on a pan. Separate the pieces before serving.

Nutrition Facts Per Serving: Calories 152 | fat 14 g | Carbohydrates 6 g | Protein 2 g

26. Warm Lentil salad

Prep time: 10 mins, Cook time: 0 min, Servings: 2

Ingredients

- 150g dried lentils
- 400ml of Vegetable bouillon, yeast-free
- Half lemon
- 2 cloves of garlic
- 1 onion
- 1 pepper or capsicum
- 4 tomatoes, skinned
- 1-inch ginger
- 1 courgette or zucchini
- A handful of coriander or basil
- Sprinkle of seeds
- Coconut oil

Instructions

- Start by simmering the lentils with a half-squeezed lemon in a vegetable stockpot. Simmer for around 30 minutes; if required, add more stock to keep the mixture from boiling dry.

- The onion should next be gently sautéed in coconut oil until transparent. The only things that may render coconut oil toxic are heat, light, and air. Even if you don't have coconut oil, you may steam fry using olive oil.

- Before incorporating the peppers, courgette, and garlic, the onion should first soften. Don't let everything go too mushy; everything should still be slightly crisp. Cook the tomatoes for a few minutes or until they are tender.

- You're finished! To taste, you must season the lentils, herbs, and seeds.

Nutrition Facts Per Serving: Calories 343|fat 12 g | Carbohydrate 45 g| Protein 9 g

---

27. Herbal Chamomile Health Tonic

Prep time: 05 mins, Cook time: 20 mins, Servings: 4

Ingredients

- 4 cups of boiling water
- 6 bags of chamomile tea
- 2 tsp of grated fresh ginger
- 4 slices of lemon
- 2-4 tsp of honey
- 2 sprigs rosemary

Instructions

- Combined with boiling water in a sizable heatproof dish are ginger, honey, lemon, and rosemary. Stirring often, steep for 20 minutes. Push the tea bags through a fine-mesh sieve to remove as much liquid as possible.

Nutrition Facts Per Serving: Calories 6 | fat 0 g | Carbohydrates 1 g | Protein 0.1 g

28. Coleslaw Zing

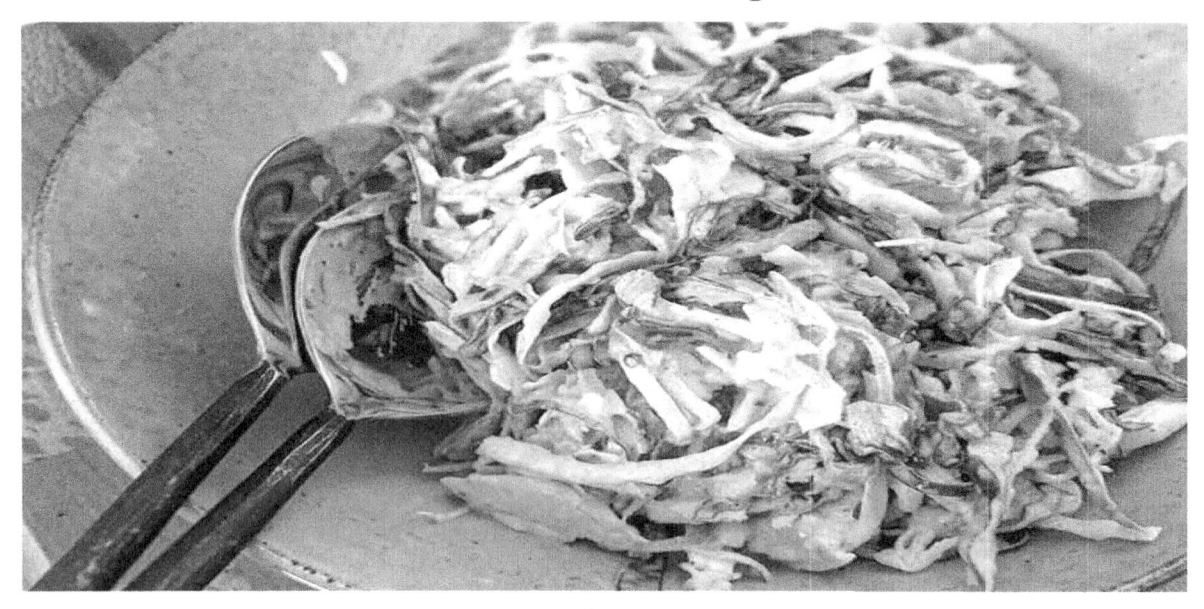

Prep time: 15 mins, Cook time: 0 min, Servings: 2

Ingredients

- 1/2 red cabbage
- 1/2 green cabbage
- 1 carrot
- 1 courgette
- 1/2 lime
- Handful of parsley
- 1 chili, small (optional)
- 2 tbsp of olive/ Udo's Choice/avocado oil
- Himalayan salt

Instructions

- Thinly sliced or grated vegetables such as cabbage, carrots, and courgettes should be used.
- Mix the parsley, chili, lime juice, salt, and oil in a bowl.
- To serve, wait till it has cooled.

Nutrition Facts Per Serving: Calories 305|fat 12.1 g | Carbohydrate 23 g| Protein 11 g

29. Broad Beans Salad with Turmeric Tomatoes

Prep time: 25 mins, Cook time: 10 min, Servings: 2

Ingredients

- 5 tbsp of coconut oil/olive oil
- 85g of broad beans
- ½ sliced onion
- 1 handful of cherry tomatoes
- Pinch of Himalayan salt or sea
- 100g of new potatoes, sliced
- 1 tsp of turmeric
- 1 handful each of basil, parsley, and chives, all chopped

Instructions

- Start by cooking the beans and broad onion in two tablespoons of coconut oil for around two minutes. If you don't have coconut oil, you can use olive oil, but I advise against it since it's the only secure cooking oil.
- Before serving, let the beans and onion cool down a bit.
- The tomatoes should be sliced in half, seasoned with salt and oil, and then placed on a counter to cool.
- The young potatoes are then parboiled. Add the turmeric and bring the mixture to a boil in a pot. After eight minutes of boiling, drain. To produce wholesome, chunky chip slices, fry them in more coconut oil for five minutes.
- Before serving, drizzle some olive oil over the dish and sprinkle on some salt. Potatoes, broad beans, and tomatoes are combined with herbs.

Nutrition Facts Per Serving: Calories 248|fat 12 g | Carbohydrate 35 g| Protein 17 g

30. Crispy Roasted Chickpeas

Prep Time: 5 mins, Cook Time: 20 mins, Servings 1-1/2

Ingredients

- 1-1/2 cups chickpeas drained
- Olive oil for drizzling
- Sea salt
- paprika

Instructions

- Put parchment paper on the baking sheet after preheating the oven to 425° F.
- Spread the chickpeas out on the cloth to drain them. Skins that have fallen off should be discarded.
- On the baking sheet, mix the dry chickpeas with a little bit of oil & salt.
- Because ovens vary, roast for 20 to 30 minutes or until roasted and crispy; if your beans aren't crispy, cook them longer until they are.
- When using, remove from the oven and combine with your desired seasonings while the chickpeas are still warm.
- Chickpeas that have been toasted should be stored in a covered container at 25 C. It is advised to use them within two days.

Nutrition Facts Per Serving: Calories 348|fat 4.6 g | Carbohydrate 53 g| Protein 13.7 g

31. Cooked Lentils

Prep Time: 5 mins, Cook Time: 20 mins, Serves 4 to 6

Ingredients

- Cooked Lentils
- 1 cup uncooked green lentils
- Water

Lemon-Herb Dressing

- 3 tbsp of lemon juice
- 1 tbsp of olive oil
- 1 tsp of sea salt
- ¼ tsp of Dijon mustard
- Black pepper freshly ground
- 1/2 cup chopped parsley
- Red chili flakes

Instructions

- In a medium saucepan, combine the lentils and water. Simmer for 20 minutes. If the potatoes are tender but not mashed, simmer them for 17 to 20 minutes with the lid on and the heat down. Take the water out and let it cool. Any recipe that calls for cooked lentils may utilize them.
- Add the cooked lentils to a small mixing bowl. Combine the fresh lemon juice, salt, oil, mustard, and pepper in a large mixing bowl. Add the parsley and red chili flakes, if desired. Serve as a dish or store in the refrigerator for five days.

Nutrition Facts Per Serving: Calories 285|fat 3.5 g | Carbohydrate 45 g| Protein 9.8 g

32. Homemade Applesauce

Prep Time: 15 mins, Cook Time: 30 mins, Servings 8

Ingredients

- 4 pounds of chopped and peeled apples
- 2 tbsp of apple vinegar
- ⅓ cup of water
- 1 tsp of apple pie spice
- Sea salt

Instructions

- Mix the apples, apple cider vinegar, and water in a big pot or Dutch oven. Cook the apples for approximately 4 minutes on low heat, stirring often.

- For 10 minutes, simmer with a cover over low heat. When the apples are incredibly soft and starting to break apart, uncover, toss in the salt and apple pie spice, then cover once more and simmer for 10 to 20 minutes.

- When the apples are at the proper consistency, please turn off the heat and mash them with a potato masher (note: avoid using a metal masher on ceramic, non-stick, or enameled cast-iron pots). Use a silicone masher or a bowl to mash the apples. Pulse the applesauce in a food processor for a smoother texture.

Nutrition Facts Per Serving: Calories 348|fat 12 g | Carbohydrate 57 g| Protein 12 g

Conclusion

It doesn't matter whether you've had a history of chronic inflammation; eating in a manner that reduces inflammation is always a good idea. Eating in a way that reduces inflammation is not just a fad, it's a lifestyle choice that will, in the long run, improve your well-being, health, and overall quality of life. A diet like these benefits everyone, but in my experience, it is beneficial for those dealing with ongoing health problems and inflammation.

You will start to feel better when you eat in this manner. It is the opinion of Dr. Scanniello that "patients may experience reduced bloating, gastrointestinal discomfort, and pains." Alterations to your diet may also cause you to experience a shift in your mental state and emotions.

If you have a health concern, you shouldn't expect to see results quickly; depending on the circumstances, it might take about a month and a half to see the long-term or short-term benefits.

If you follow the anti-inflammatory diet to a T and are aware of which foods to include in your diet and which ones to exclude, there are no significant adverse side effects.

If processed foods and dairy products make up most of your current diet, you may experience some discomfort throughout the transition period. Because of this, you'll have to put in much more work and time while cooking your meals, and you won't be able to indulge in any processed foods while following this technique.

A diet that takes an anti-inflammatory strategy involves consuming many foods that have been shown to lower inflammation and restricting your intake of foods that take the opposite approach. However, one of the best things about the diet is that it gives you a broad range of meal options and a lot of leeway in terms of flexibility.

If you want to bring more structure to the way you eat, the Mediterranean diet can be an excellent choice for you to consider. There is a lot of overlap between the two diets since they both emphasize eating whole fruits, vegetables, and whole grains. An anti-inflammatory and alkaline diet may halt disease advancement, reduce the need for medication, and protect joints from further damage.

Made in United States
North Haven, CT
20 February 2023